"Brave and elegiac...Ultimately it's a story of what it is to love someone with mental illness." *Editor's Choice, Bookseller*

"(Simpson) vividly and thoughtfully unpicks the circumstances in which she and her sisters were raised ... a study in gender oppression." *Times Literary Supplement*

"Mixes the coolness of her journalistic training with the subjective pain of loss." *James Robertson*

"A deeply engaging, courageous and human work." *Graeme Macrae Burnet*

"This book's secret weapon ... is the remarkable voice that fires from the page to the heart with no hesitation at all. Just wonderful." *Janice Galloway*

"Simpson reconstructs a complicated portrait of the past with tenderness and unsparing detail." *The List*

"A very powerful and moving read." *Literary Sofa*

Praise for *Truestory*:

"Moving but never mawkish, and ultimately hopeful, a sympathetic portrait of ... autism." *Sunday Mirror*

"Sharply observed...a terrific read." *The Herald*

"Vivid and empathetic." *Lothian Life*

"I giggled and welled up at different times ... prepare yourself for the roller-coaster journey." *Novelicious*

"Vivid, perceptive and acute." *James Robertson*

"Captivating, poignant and vivid." *Dundee University Review of the Arts*

One Body

A retrospective

Catherine Simpson

Saraband

Published by Saraband
3 Clairmont Gardens
Glasgow, G3 7LW
www.saraband.net

ISBN: 9781913393342

1 2 3 4 5 6 7 8 9 10

Printed and bound in Great Britain by Clays Ltd, Elcograf S.p.A.

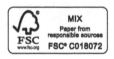

This book is for Cello,
beside me every step of the way

(like Billy Connolly's Mary!)

One

I was born at milking time on a dairy farm, which must have been a nuisance. I would learn later that nothing got in the way of milking and it was never acceptable to be a nuisance.

Nurse Steele attended my mother, who was in bed in the best sitting room; afterwards, the doctor, who had arrived in time for the birth, picked his way across the dark farmyard, through the puddles and over the cobbles, to the cowshed to inform my dad, 'Another girl!'

It was late October back in sixty-three, and as Frankie Valli might have said, 'Oh, What a Night'. Being farmers, they must have wanted a boy, but seeing as I weighed a decent eight pounds and had ten fingers and ten toes, they got what they were given.

My mother could not breastfeed and I refused bottled milk (another nuisance on a dairy farm), so legend has it she fed me 'liquidised sandwiches'.

At three months, before any of my vaccinations, I got whooping cough and she sat up night after night with me in front of the kitchen range, waiting for the 'whoop' between the coughs, thinking I had drawn my last breath. Over the years I was told every now and then, 'You nearly died, you did; think on.'

My mother also told me she had fallen downstairs when she was pregnant with me and remarked more than once, 'I didn't make such a good job of you.'

One way or another I used up a lot of my mother's patience before I was even old enough to remember.

I was not raised with permission to be ill – as I grew up, illness was barely tolerated.

Doctors' surgeries were for inoculations. Hospitals were for dealing with accidents, with the occasional stitch or a plaster cast. For years our farmhouse did not contain a first-aid kit and the only medication we had was a bottle of orange-flavoured Junior Aspirin on the top shelf in the kitchen to shut us up if we felt 'poorly' and a tin of sticky pink Germolene for cuts and grazes.

One of my most prized possessions was a 'nurse's bag' I got for my eighth birthday, which contained a pretend syringe and a hammer for 'knocking knees'. But I knew no one who worked in the medical profession; I was more familiar with the veterinary surgeon. We often watched the vet at work on the farm, injecting animals and calving cows. We also watched the artificial insem-inator, the AI, at work in his enormous rubber apron, taking a straw of bull semen and sticking his arm up to his armpit inside a cow. This was mysterious but also normal. So normal that when we played in the muddy banks of the pond, we shoved our hands in deep, brought them out with a 'plop' and shouted, 'I'm the AI!'

At our village primary school, Mrs Darlington had 'magic cream', a cream that took away all pain, stopped all aches and cured all illness. I imagine it was Savlon, but for years I believed it said 'magic cream' on the tube. I longed for magic cream, but I never got any because I never had any ailments.

When one of the boys broke his leg tripping over a slab in the playground, magic cream was not applied; instead he was put at the front of the classroom with his leg propped up on a chair and a wet paper towel on top until home time.

Children who were ill were exotic. Illness made them worthy of fuss (a chair at the front, a wet paper towel). Illness made them special.

One girl in the village said she saw pink elephants dance around her bedroom walls during a fever, and I was fascinated and envious of what sounded like her own Disney film. When another girl was sent for speech therapy because she said 'bastick' instead of 'basket', I decided to develop a stutter, until I got home and my mother barked, 'Talk properly!'

In our dressing-up box, my sisters and I had a pair of Victorian wire-framed spectacles. We took turns sitting on the wall at the front of the farmhouse, the world swimming through the lenses, waiting for the occasional car to pass by in the hope that the driver would think we were intelligent and interesting enough to need glasses. In fact, I *was* short-sighted and did need glasses, but nobody noticed until I was eight and had a school eye test, by which time I could no longer read the blackboard.

NHS spectacles came in pink, blue or tortoiseshell. I refused the pink because they were too 'albino rabbit', and the tortoiseshell ones were for clever boys with short back and sides who did their own experiments, so I ended up with the pale blue.

Glasses were a blow for a child; it would be years before they became stylish. You were a 'Speccy Four-Eyes' or a 'Mr Magoo' – a cartoon character who blundered around half-blind. My uncle told me, 'Boys don't make passes at girls who wear glasses.' This was the same uncle who said, 'Pink, pink, makes the boys wink', which may have been another reason I rejected the pink frames. Glasses, it turned out, did not make me more interesting or intelligent and were definitely not exotic; indeed, there was something sad and lonely about them.

I refused to wear my glasses and ran the bed castors over them several times. They were presumably designed for this eventuality because they bent into the carpet but never broke.

At high school, my two best friends and I got matching silver-framed glasses. On catching sight of us, the deranged biology teacher yelled, 'What are you doing in my classroom glinting like a row of Nazis?'

No, glasses were not special or exotic and mostly I hid them in my pocket, preferring the world to be fuzzy.

One Body

I got contact lenses at sixteen, as soon as the optician would prescribe them. Sometimes I would forget to remove them at night and for a glorious moment on waking I would think my sight had been restored; the trees had leaves! Then, with a sinking heart I would feel the terrible grating and have to drag the lenses off my dried-up eyeballs like peeling Elastoplast off a burn.

I resented wearing glasses because they made my eyes look smaller – having big eyes was something people had remarked on all my life, *Ooh, big brown eyes!*, as though I had done something right when I chose them.

Childhood illnesses were a disappointment. When my little sister Tricia was lying on the sofa red hot and covered in chickenpox from head to toe, I got one spot on my belly.

Baby teeth rotted out of our heads; that was no big deal. Toothache was as normal as, well, toothache. Wobbly baby teeth were got rid of by eating an apple or chewing on a toffee, or if that didn't work, my grandad would threaten to tie the tooth to an open door and slam it – a suggestion that made me wobble loose teeth secretly until that last bit of stretchy flesh gave way and I tasted blood.

Inexplicably, our 1970s dentist extracted the odd healthy second tooth, leaving permanent yawning gaps. He used laughing gas, which a cousin complained smelled of farts and polos, after which we were sent on our bikes to the Post Office for the cure: an ice cream.

A day off school ill was rare enough to be mythical. I remember my dumb surprise when a friend's mother said she would not be in school that day because she had 'a sniffle'. I glimpsed my friend lying in bed surrounded by crumpled tissues and reeking of something called Olbas Oil, and wondered: what strange world is this?

Car sickness was treated with barley sugar, a stomach ache with dry bread, nettle stings with dock leaves, splinters you nibbled out with your teeth. Children did not get headaches. When I came home from primary school and told my mum I had not been able to see the blackboard for flashing lights, she remarked, 'Oh, you've had a migraine, like Uncle John', and never mentioned it again.

As a child, I found sick people in books alluring because illness apparently made you lovable. Cousin Helen in *What Katy Did* was sweet-natured, generous, wise and gentle, and lay on the sofa all day with ruffles on her nightie, laughing merrily or smiling beatifically, 'half an angel already', like Beth March from *Little Women*, who was 'very patient and bore her pain uncomplainingly'. I did not envy Beth her scarlet fever like I envied Jo's writing, Amy's ringlets and Meg's handsome husband, but being on her death-bed certainly made her popular. And then there was Cathy, the consumptive, pale and beautiful girl who faded away with grace to be buried on the moor and send Heathcliff mad with grief in *Wuthering Heights*.

'Invalids', it seemed, were the centre of attention for doing not much more than being fragile and beautiful.

But I was brought up to believe that in real life there was no time or room for Illness and as a middle-aged woman I still dreaded making a fuss and wasting the doctor's time. In my GP's surgery was a notice: *Do you have skin tags that cause pain? Because if so the necessary minor surgical procedure can be carried out here.* When I saw this, I blinked; if I had skin tags that caused pain, I cut them off with nail scissors.

Two

I am in the outer waiting room. Waiting.

I make notes because, as a writer, you never know when you might need the *exact* details of a breast clinic waiting room.

Local radio plays: '...*and get your early bird tickets to ... physical injuries compensation ... for all your energy needs...*' The emphatic adverts and jingles segue into pop songs, but the volume is quiet out here, beyond the safety of the reception desk.

My husband, Cello, is reading, *If on a Winter's Night a Traveller.* I was going to come to today's appointment alone, but a friend said no, take Cello.

More notes. I squeak on the wipe-clean banquette as I swivel to gaze at a plastic bonsai beside a tub marked: *Donations to Breast Cancer Charity. Thank you.*

I am the first appointment, but sunshine already streams through the glass doors. It is 1 August and we are in the middle of a heatwave. Heatwaves hold such *suspense* – something about their brooding stillness.

A smiling woman appears in black trousers and a patterned top.

'Catherine? Can you come through?'

I assume an 'I'm listening' pose: hands on lap, head slightly cocked, handbag tucked by my feet.

She introduces herself as Lizzie, a breast care nurse.

My appointment letter inviting me here today said the results of my mammogram a month ago were 'unclear'; they did not say they were 'abnormal', so I am confident everything will be resolved quickly.

'So, this is the area we are concerned about.'

Lizzie turns her computer screen to face us. On it is the shape of my right breast in black. At the upper outer edge is what looks like a silver shooting star; a far-distant meteor burning bright in the night sky. Lizzie outlines it with the end of her biro and Cello and I lean forward in unison. It is quite pretty, glowing, too airy to appear significant.

Can something made of light be dangerous?

Contradictory thoughts collide: 'You've called me back for *this* shiny little thing?' and 'Oh, so there *is* something.'

But the image is crystal clear. I have been fooled; the mammogram is not 'unclear', as in 'out-of-focus', but 'unclear' as in 'we don't know what this is...'.

Lizzie explains that the area is white on the mammogram because it is denser than the rest of the breast. She asks me to go behind the curtain and undress from the waist up. I lie down behind the rattling curtain that hangs too close to the bed and she examines me – tapping and circling – but even though she knows where the 'shooting star' is, she cannot feel anything. No lump. Nothing. I regain confidence; yes, this will be sorted out in no time.

I am in the inner waiting room. Waiting.

I am alone. Cello has been sent back to the outer waiting room. In my notebook I write, 'Inner sanctum of the breast clinic'. This waiting room is pinker, more female, more middle-aged. A handmade patchwork quilt hangs on a lilac wall. There are dogeared copies of *Which?*, *Woman & Home* and *Celebrate*.

A sign says: *Please Turn off Your Mobile Phone*, which seems cruel in this isolating room.

Here the quality of the waiting is different. Out there it was low-key, low-energy waiting, clock-watching, let's-fill-my-notebook-so-as-not-to-waste-time waiting. But now I am on my own, things have taken an unexpected turn, and the waiting is high-alert waiting.

I have been singled out. I learned as a child that to be 'singled out' was never a good thing. To be singled out meant to be picked on, to be bullied, to be blamed or to be shamed.

I remind myself of a cow separated from the herd, corralled alone, ready to go to the abattoir. Perhaps this is not such an unusual thought if you were raised on a dairy farm. I remember the frightened expressions of cows when they found themselves unexpectedly apart. Singled out.

Through the window, the sky is blue. High on a neighbouring tenement, a self-set buddleia takes root, leggy, flowering, defiant.

What matters to you? asks a poster.

What matters to me is getting out of here.

I pace the room. *Laugh More, Worry Less!* declares the cover of *Woman & Home. Too Busy? Learn the Art of Saying No.*

I have never been good at saying 'no'. I perch on a chair and go through the motions of flicking through the magazine. Maybe it will give me some tips. I am still blindly flicking when a woman in a blue uniform leans round the door.

'Catherine? Can you come through?'

Another mammogram. *Lean in … a bit more … hold your breath.* My hair dangles in the way. She suggests I tie it up, but I don't have a hair elastic and I am struck by a devastating feeling of unpreparedness, a sinking right through my core.

I am an amateur at this.

I have been lured here under false pretences. The letter said this appointment was a *routine second stage of screening*, that *1 in 20 women were invited back* and that *4 out of 5 women who are invited back are found not to have breast cancer.*

I believed everything would be all right because I was brought up never to be a nuisance and having breast cancer would be nothing if not a nuisance.

The mammographer sticks the nib of her pen through a blue latex glove, rips off the cuff and hands it to me to use as a hair tie.

She is capable, confident, in charge. I am not.

An ultrasound. I lie on the bed and the nurse squirts my left breast with a clear jelly. It is icy cold, and I shudder. It is also the wrong breast. 'I think it's this one,' I say, and we laugh.

My only other ultrasounds were when I was pregnant with my daughters, Nina and Lara, twenty-three and twenty years ago. Then there was excitement and anticipation in the room. A warm buzz. The screen was turned to face us so we could gaze at the baby's heartbeat, its floating lava-lamp limbs. Cello was with me. We were excited to see something growing inside me, relieved and grateful, hardly believing it.

After both antenatal ultrasounds we left with a photograph – a blurry black and white image of what looked like a moon landing – an image I studied for clues about who this person would be. An image I framed both times and put on the television, much to my dad's consternation. He was a farmer used to delivering calves, but he shook his head at my insides being on display in the living room.

I was offered only one ultrasound with each baby but wanted more. 'Why,' asked a midwife, 'what do you want to see?'

'The future,' I said.

But today I am not so sure.

Today the ultrasound technician turns the screen away. She moves the hand scanner slowly over the top of my breast, pressing hard, as I lie with my right arm above my head. The nurse stands at the

Two

other side of the bed and chats. What do I do for a living? I tell them I'm a writer; that I have a memoir coming out soon. 'We've all got a book in us, haven't we?' says the nurse and the ultrasound technician nods, 'If only we had the time to write it.'

I am in a vulnerable position and say nothing.

The ultrasound technician peers at her screen. 'There's something there that's different from everything around it,' she says to the screen, 'and I'm concerned about one of the lymph nodes.' I try to catch her eye, giving her the chance to mention benign lumps and cysts, but she looks away and says, 'I'll get the consultant.'

The nurse grimaces and squeezes my hand.

The ultrasound technician disappears and a small, bespectacled middle-aged woman strides in, unnervingly wrapping a plastic disposable apron over her blue dress as she walks.

'We'll need a biopsy. Shall we do it now?'

At this moment, lying flat on my back, half naked, I get the first inkling of terror. Life is going wrong, picking up speed on an unexpected detour, and I cannot stop it.

I nod and turn away. My teeth chatter. I have heard horror stories of breast biopsies, but I've learned over the years that what I dread seeks me out.

I will have a 'core biopsy' – a large, hollow needle will be inserted to remove samples of tissue.

'This may sting a bit,' the consultant says. 'It may nip a little.'

She injects local anaesthetic and cuts the skin to insert the biopsy needle. She uses the ultrasound to guide the needle. She warns me there will be a loud clunk. There is: KER-CHUNK! And pain sears through my breast. Tears leak down the sides of my face, but I can't wipe them away because one arm is stuck above my head and the other is clinging to the nurse. They need another two samples. I shake my head and tears splash cold against my nose. I am good with pain, but not this.

She injects more anaesthetic and takes two further samples. The pain fades but with each sample comes another unnerving KER-CHUNK! She places a 'metal marker' in my body to mark the location. 'It won't set off airport scanners or anything,' she says. I imagine her slotting in a supermarket trolley token, but in fact I learn later on Google that the markers are titanium and smaller than a sesame seed.

'What is the chance of this biopsy coming back as nothing to worry about?' I ask.

The consultant grimaces and shakes her head. I realise no one has said 'don't worry' since I got here. My stomach turns, my skin chills and the world decisively shifts.

The nurse avoids my eye and squeezes my hand even harder.

'Is it stress that has done this to me?' I ask. The consultant shrugs. 'We don't really know. Probably genetics?'

'But ... I've got a book coming out ... I've got a wedding to go to ... I haven't got time for this.' I do a sort-of-laugh. Nobody else laughs. They close the wound with paper stitches and a dressing and give me instructions about caring for it, but I don't take in a word.

'What are you doing for the rest of the day?' asks the consultant.

'My VAT return.'

She pulls that face again. 'Maybe do something else.'

I have no memory of getting off the bed, of putting on my Kate Bush T-shirt or gathering my stuff. Months later I realise I have never worn that T-shirt since and probably never will.

I am taken for another mammogram to check the metal marker is in the right place.

But still the word 'cancer' has never been spoken.

I go to the outer waiting room, where the sun still pours through the window and Cello is deep in his book.

'They think there might be something,' I say, and signal for him to follow me.

Afterwards, he tells me I came out smiling, which must be my dread of being a nuisance again; always trying to smooth things over, play things down.

I arrived at the clinic that morning believing I would be one of the *4 out of 5* who would leave with nothing to worry about, but now there was a door with my name on it. Literally. As I am taken back into Nurse Lizzie's room, she slips a piece of paper into a slot on the door: 'Occupied. Catherine Simpson.'

'That's a lot to take in,' she says.

I gaze at her. It is both a lot, and nothing. No one has said I have cancer. Nothing has been spelled out.

'Shall I go through it again?' she asks.

'Yes,' Cello and I answer together.

She starts talking, but again it is as though I am plunged into the middle of a conversation having missed the beginning. I hear, 'Young women with cancer…' and I ask, 'Is that me?' and when she says an emphatic 'Oh, yes!' I realise she thinks I am asking if I am young to have cancer, not whether I have cancer at all. She continues, 'Many of the ladies we deal with are in their seventies and eighties.'

It is like watching a flickering screen, a wildly speeded-up film where images flash past with no time to make sense of them. I am suspended in front of chaos. My breathing has gone shallow, but if I start to breathe properly it will mean accepting cancer as my new reality.

'You need to lie down,' says Lizzie.

It takes me a moment to realise she is talking to Cello. His face is drained, yellow and sweating. 'I'll be all right,' he says. He bends double on his seat.

But Lizzie insists. 'Lie down. The last husband who did this landed on the floor and I couldn't get him up.'

She helps Cello to the bed where an hour and a half before I was being examined behind the rattling curtain. He lies down and she puts a damp paper towel on his head and a cushion under his feet.

I start laughing, then crying. Then both; laughing as I wipe away tears. Isn't this typical? We have a family joke: I am a 'Tough Lancashire Lass' and Cello is an 'Italian Mummy's Boy'. Fifteen years ago we both had accidents a fortnight apart on an artificial ski slope. I broke my arm in two places trying to avoid a Brownie pack and got myself and my two primary school-aged children off the slope and removed my skis before asking for help. Whereas when Cello slipped and noticed his little finger at a funny angle, he fainted, out cold, face-planted on the ski matting, permanently scarring his forehead in the process, before being stretchered off the nursery slope.

I continue half-laughing, half-crying, drying my eyes with the back of my hand, but Lizzie does not laugh. Apparently, husbands do this a lot.

Eventually Cello sits up and Lizzie explains the biopsy samples will be sent to pathology for analysis. The results will take twelve days. They used to take a week, but due to staff shortages it now takes up to a fortnight. She arranges an appointment in twelve days' time, warning that if the results are delayed it will be postponed.

As she taps on her keyboard, I text an old school friend, Carole, who knows I am at the breast clinic.

'I may have breast cancer. I have to wait 12 days to find out.'

An answer pings straight back: *'Fuck! Fuck! Fucking hell! and Fuck! again for good measure.'*

The perfect response.

Two

Shortly after, Cello and I emerge, wordless, into the noon-day heat, from this ugly building – a building I entered well and left sick. I have taken my health for granted. I do not feel like a patient. I do not feel like a sick person. I do not feel like someone with a disease that requires immediate treatment. We head down to the higgledy-piggledy car park and into a different world.

A twelve-day wait in diagnostic limbo. Medical no man's land. Twelve days, twelve nights, twelve evenings, twelve mornings, twelve showers, twelve breakfasts, twelve lunches, twelve dinners. Twelve endless interminable days of not knowing. Twelve terrifying sleepless nights of fearing the worst. Two hundred and eighty-eight hours; seventeen thousand, two hundred and eighty minutes, each one a lifetime.

I decided not to tell my daughters and elderly father until I knew for sure as I still hoped it was a mistake. There was no lump, after all. No pain. If it had not been for a routine mammogram, my life would still be sailing along nicely, but then I would recall the consultant's grim expression and the definite shake of her head and go cold from head to foot.

I had Schrödinger's cancer: both there and not there, both growing and non-existent.

My mind was sharp. I had a sense of urgency to clear the decks – to be *ready*. My senses had switched to 'super-alert' in a height-ened world.

At a friend's fiftieth birthday party that weekend I said noth-ing, not wanting to be the spectre at the feast. I ate, drank and acted merry, then slipped away. Outwardly I was a Beryl Cook painting, inwardly an Edvard Munch woodcut: externally enjoy-ing the party, internally screaming in terror.

I fell back on making sense of things with words and headed up my notebook: *The Twelve Days of Not Knowing*, but no words came.

The world had become an uncanny place, at once familiar and unfamiliar. Home was not homely any more – it was strange and unsettling – and I no longer felt safe there because I no longer felt safe anywhere.

When the sense of urgency deserted me on day four, I forced myself to keep busy: folding washing, cooking, shopping, tasks to distract me from the terror.

And terror it was.

A terror that descended cell by cell throughout my body, chilled my skin, tightened my stomach; it stilled me to a paralysis, which I fought by going through the motions of more chores. A terror like a dead weight that slowed my body as it speeded up my mind with panic-stricken thoughts whirring, ungraspable and wild. A terror that jolted me awake in the darkest hours of the night and kept me awake thinking about my own extinction, about being separated from my children for ever – no matter that they were now young adults. A terror of no longer being, and the world carrying on regardless.

I stared into the dark in bed at night, peering into the future to imagine my own death, unable to turn away from what we usually avoid.

I did not wake Cello because then there would have been two of us helpless and sleepless. Once he woke and found me crying. He put his arms round me, but I was still alone; the glowing shooting star was in me, not in anyone else.

'It's worse for your loved ones than it is for you,' I was told several times, but in the middle of the night cancer made me feel startlingly and breathtakingly alone.

Two

For the full twelve days our elder daughter Nina had her fiancé, Shane, visiting from America. I said nothing, not wanting to spoil their time together. Our other daughter, Lara, was at Camp America in New Jersey. We FaceTimed Lara several times during the twelve days and it took a monumental effort to look cheerful and normal and not to sob with fear and despair.

On Shane's second-to-last night, two days before the test results, the four of us went out to eat. It was getting harder to act normal. I was standing near a cliff edge watching the ground crumble towards my feet. After the meal, Nina and Shane left us to finish the wine, and ten minutes later Cello and I wandered home. The Edinburgh Fringe Festival was in full swing and as we passed the Playhouse Theatre, we noticed that the comedian Frankie Boyle – controversial, pessimistic Frankie Boyle – was about to come on stage. I gazed at his name up in lights over the Playhouse doors and knew I *needed* to see Frankie Boyle; at that moment, nothing and nobody could help me as much as Frankie Boyle. The box office staff told us there were seats available up in the gods.

'Come on,' I said.

He strode on stage, a Viking in a C&A suit. 'I hope you're not a sensitive crowd,' he said, 'because this is going to be a cancer-heavy hour.' I started laughing. I *knew* this was a good idea. I saw Cello gauging my reaction before he started laughing too. There were more cancer jokes. All funny. It felt good to laugh at this thing that was holding me hostage. It felt joyful and trium-phant to be part of this crowd. When Frankie Boyle harangued a man in the audience – 'Oh you're lucky, aren't you? Bet you're the type who gets to your target weight at Weight Watchers the week you're diagnosed with cancer' – it was as if Frankie Boyle had written the script especially for me, considering I had recently lost a stone at a slimming club.

We walked home still laughing, and Cello said, 'We can't complain. We knew what we were in for.'

At home I searched my bookshelves for Frankie Boyle's autobiography, *My Shit Life So Far.* I needed his nihilistic take on life. If life meant nothing, then death meant nothing, and this experience meant nothing.

I didn't know if Frankie Boyle was giving me bravery or bravado, but whatever it was he was providing a temporary shelter.

I fantasised about the results being clear and pictured us celebrating with real champagne in real champagne flutes. I could hear it, smell it, taste it. I imagined the stories I could tell about this terrible twelve days.

But I couldn't hold on to this optimism, and the afternoon before the results I Googled 'metastatic cancer' and felt the world sway.

Not telling people had become a burden.

On the eve of results day, Cello and I were in a local café. The proprietor strode over, a smiling, bluff, mine-host type of a man. He pulled his jacket around his paunch and made conversation as his chef prepared our pizzas. He told a story about a couple he knew who got married then discovered the wife had cancer, so they split up. He threw his hands in the air and did a short laugh, looking for a response.

We gazed at him, wordless.

He smiled uncertainly, readjusted his jacket and went to check on the pizzas.

When Cello and I returned to the clinic, we were both shown into the 'inner sanctum' waiting room. By now I had realised that this cancer thing (if that's what it was) would include much waiting – but no waiting was more excruciating than this last hour.

I was half an hour early. I couldn't concentrate at home, so I came to the clinic to be physically closer to the results. Every time footsteps marched towards the door, I held my breath, then slumped as they marched past. When voices drifted along the corridor I sat up, listening like a dog on high alert, until they faded away again.

This time I could not face making notes or leafing through magazines. I had no brave face left to put on. All I could do was gaze at the floor in misery. My appointment time of 2.30pm came and went. 2.35pm, 2.40pm. Someone poked their head in to say the team were often late due to traffic. I stared endlessly at my watch. 2.45pm, 2.50pm. I began to wonder if I would be in limbo forever. After the twelve never-ending days this was the final straw.

Another middle-aged couple came into the waiting room and our terror was reflected in their faces. This woman, like me, had blow-dried her hair and applied full make-up. We sat, speechless, until I blurted out, 'This is torture,' and the man nodded, 'Yes, it is.' The woman stayed mute. Eventually she was called for her appointment, but my wait continued. 2.55pm, 3pm. Then, at last:

'Catherine? Can you come through?'

I had expected to see the hospital consultant, but it was a young woman with a blonde ponytail, who wore a badge saying 'houseman', which I learned later was a junior doctor. As I entered the room she was poring over my notes. She talked as her eyes continued to scan the page. The results were back, and she read them out, but they were in a medical jargon I did not understand.

The word 'cancer' was not used, but I gathered I needed an operation to remove what they had discovered. My mind snagged on this information.

So, it *was* cancer.

I had cancer.

I was a woman with breast cancer.

I remember nothing else of what she said and then she was gone. Fortunately, Nurse Lizzie was there again with a booklet, *Understanding Breast Cancer in Women*.

She laid it on the desk, drawing asterisks beside 'Invasive lobular breast cancer', then 'Stage 1' then 'Grade 2' then 'ER Positive' and 'PR Positive'.

I was overwhelmed by both the blunt force of the cancer diagnosis and these incomprehensible details.

Lizzie explained I would need a lumpectomy to cut away the tumour, an operation for which there was a six-week wait.

She could see I was lost and tried to reassure me, saying, 'There are ladies we treat who are still walking around…' she waved the booklet for emphasis, '…*twenty years* after treatment.'

I was fifty-four and not reassured; my mother died of cancer at seventy-four and it had felt too young. Anyway, my father was ninety-two and living independently – having a long-lived parent makes anything less seem like short change.

I asked about the lymph nodes – remembering the ultrasound technician's concern about one of them. Lizzie explained we would not know whether the cancer had passed through the lymph nodes and possibly spread until after the lumpectomy, during which several lymph nodes would also be removed for analysis.

I was crushed that although I had a definite cancer diagnosis, the wait for clarity continued.

Much as Euro Disney had taught me to queue.

And being a civil servant had taught me to form-fill.

Cancer would teach me to wait.

Three

When I left home aged nineteen for a job fifty miles away in a town where I knew nobody, I had barely seen a doctor in my life. I had never made a doctor's appointment and knew nothing about having to register. Painkillers had barely been used at home and had been eked out – halving them, quartering them – but period cramps finally drove me to the doctor's in this new town to ask for contraceptive pills in the hope that they would ease the pain.

'You can't just walk off the street into a doctor's surgery!' barked the receptionist.

It had taken courage to ask for help with the taboo subjects of periods and the pill, when I barely had the words to do so, and to be rebuffed at the first hurdle was devastating. The receptionist glared through the glass, slapped a registration form down on the counter and wordlessly slid it towards me.

I retreated humiliated to the chemist next door, where I burst into tears and the assistants commiserated, shaking their heads, 'Those receptionists can be like that!'

It was a pity that my attempt to get the pill was a failure because three months later I was pregnant; an unwanted teenage pregnancy by a man who was not only my boss and older than me but married. A man I thought I was in love with, when I was probably just lonely from leaving work every evening, watching my colleagues return to their families, as I went home to a barely furnished council flat, surrounded above, below and on each side by strangers, with hours alone stretching ahead.

He drove me back to the same doctor's to register so I could ask for a pregnancy test because over-the-counter tests were not available then. I explained my symptoms to the doctor: late period, extreme tiredness, occasional nausea, and he asked, 'Have you ever been pregnant before?', which was like being doused with icy water. He told me to leave a urine sample at the practice, then 'ring in a few days' for the pregnancy test results.

According to my diary, back at my flat, alone, I *sobbed until my head ached*.

I waited day after day for the pregnancy test results, phoning the doctor's surgery from various telephone boxes around town. *No, nothing back from the lab yet, please ring again tomorrow.*

The third day was a Saturday, and I was back at the farm. I could not use the telephone in the farmhouse because it was too public, so I walked to the local phone box. It was lashing with rain, as though the world was as upset as me. I headed outside, my dad giving me a quizzical look, as I pretended it was normal to go for a walk in a howling gale. I rang from the phone box I used to shelter in to wait for the school bus only a year or two before.

No, nothing back from the lab yet, please ring again on Monday.

On the sixth day, I stood with my fingers crossed in a phone box outside a pub called The Junction and I was told *the test is positive*, and the lyrics of Squeeze's 'Up the Junction' went round and round in my head.

My boss stood outside the phone box, leaning on the heavy door to keep it open as he smoked a fag. I looked at him, said, 'It's positive', and we went into the pub for a stiff drink – which was one of the reasons we had got into this mess in the first place.

'Don't worry, Cath, we'll sort it out,' he said.

I could not tell my parents. My father was in the middle of treatment for bone cancer, horrendous chemotherapy that laid him out, retching, after each treatment, as my mother struggled to keep the farm going. An unwanted pregnancy would be the final straw. I knew my mother would be ashamed and furious; the 1960s did not reach our Lancashire village until at least the 1990s.

Three

I told the only member of my family I could. 'Get rid of it,' they said.

I told an efficient work colleague who always knew what to do.

'I know what to do,' she said, picking up the Yellow Pages and flicking through in a businesslike way. 'You need the Pregnancy Advisory Service. They do abortions.'

I told my old school friends, but they were as young and out of their depth as I was.

A married woman, a few years older than us, who was part of our conversation that particular evening, had recently discovered she was pregnant herself and said, 'There's nothing nicer than waiting for your first baby.' I burst into tears and told her the full story, and she said, 'If you want to keep it, keep it. He *has* to help you.' Hers was the only dissenting voice.

There could be no happy ending to this story.

I lay on the floor of my flat and punched myself in the stomach. An unwanted pregnancy had always seemed like the ultimate disaster – a real terror – and here it was. There was no denying this problem, no running away from it.

I had no idea about what employment, welfare or housing rights I had – in fact, it never crossed my mind that I had any. I was on my own, veering from despair that I couldn't keep the baby to determination that I would find a way. I spoke to the father of the baby when he called from another random phone box that weekend.

'I've decided to keep it.'

'Right,' he said.

The next day, when I saw him, I was back to hopelessness and had changed my mind.

'I can't do it,' I said.

'Right,' he said again. 'I was coming round to your way of thinking.'

I ran a hot bath; maybe that would wash it away like it did in films. I poured in bath oil. *Give yourself the gentle luxury of a Fenjal Crème Bath.* I hugged my knees in the bath, wishing so hard that I could rewind time. The bath did nothing except sap more energy, leaving me so exhausted I fell asleep on the living room carpet, waking up hours later in the dark.

The smell of Fenjal still knocks me sick more than thirty-five years later.

I was numb with shock, struggling through the days, dragging a heavy emptiness with me. *What shall I do?* I kept writing in my diary. *What shall I do?* I felt *dismal* with nausea and could eat nothing but curry and instant mashed potato. I felt overwhelmed physically and emotionally.

The whole country was agog that week because Margaret Thatcher's favourite minister, Cecil Parkinson, had got his secretary, Sara Keays, pregnant and, despite having previously proposed to her and promised to leave his wife, he demanded she abort the baby. She refused, and he resigned from the government. The baby girl was born with disabilities and Parkinson never met her. His resignation during the Tory Party Conference, down the road in Blackpool, was all over the newspapers as I went to the Pregnancy Advisory Service in Manchester.

To get an abortion I had to get the signature of two doctors. I told the first doctor I was nineteen but would soon be twenty, and she interrupted matter-of-factly, 'No; you are nineteen!' and she signed the form. As did the second doctor. In Great Britain, abortion is permitted on various grounds, including risk of injury to the mental health of the pregnant woman, and, although this wasn't spelled out, I sensed that mine being an unwanted 'teenage pregnancy' made it more clear-cut.

I also had to see a counsellor. I explained about my own father being ill, about how the father of the baby was older than me and married. She asked if my employer knew, and I said, 'The father is my boss.' She said, 'We're going in smaller and smaller circles', and I thought she was going to cry.

The father of the baby went to the bank and applied for a loan to pay for the termination, telling the manager he needed the money 'for repairs'.

A few days later he took the day off work and drove me to the clinic in Liverpool, telling me he was a Catholic and didn't really believe in this sort of thing, but driving onwards, anyway.

He came with me into the full-yet-silent waiting room and wrote a cheque at the small reception – a hatch in the wall – then was told he could go no further.

I was only eight weeks pregnant, but the operation still necessitated a general anaesthetic and an overnight stay in hospital. The first time for both of these things for me.

At the clinic, I shared a room with three others also in for terminations – two teenage girls and a twenty-year-old. One of the teenagers had recently fallen off her boyfriend's motorbike and had her leg in plaster. The other two had come over from Ireland – one from the Republic and the other from Northern Ireland – where abortion was illegal and would remain so for another thirty-five years, necessitating this trip to Liverpool. None of us had told our parents and neither of the Irish girls had told the fathers of their babies.

The girl from the Republic of Ireland had flown over that morning and was flying home the following morning with her brother, who had come as her support.

The Northern Irish girl had arrived alone that day on the early-morning ferry and was travelling back the following day on the late-night ferry – having to spend almost two days away from home for this medical procedure and filling the long hours before and after the operation sitting in cinemas, hairdressers and cafés.

The only person she had confided in was her parish priest, who had told her that what she was contemplating was a mortal sin and she would be 'a mental cripple for the rest of her life' if she went through with it.

We were given a rundown of what to expect by a brisk-brusque nurse and then I was first in for the operation. I remember lying on a trolley being wheeled fast along the corridor as I tried to explain they had not given me the pre-med. I remember the smiling face of a young man in scrubs looking down at me. 'Us? Forget?' and then sharp jabs in my hand. I remember watching the brisk-brusque nurse's white shoes squeaking as she marched down the corridor alongside my trolley – but how can I remember that? I was lying on the trolley – I could not have seen the nurse's shoes. Am I remembering Nurse Ratched from *One Flew Over the Cuckoo's Nest*?

I remember nothing else until I woke up back in bed, rocking from side to side, moaning, my body cramping and bleeding into a giant sanitary pad. I remember wondering who was making all the noise.

'Sssh,' the nurse said, putting her hand on my shoulder, 'lie still!'

I remember being embarrassed and curling up as quiet and still as death and listening to the other girls quietly crying around me.

By that evening we were sitting up in bed talking. The Northern Irish girl said, 'Goodbye, morning sickness, hello, periods,' and then added, 'I wanted them to baptise what came out.'

The girl with the broken leg was visited by her boyfriend dressed in full motorcycle leathers, who sat silently beside her bed, holding her hand, his head bowed.

My boss came to visit, bringing a carrier bag of chocolate bars to share out between the four of us, all desperate for sugar.

The two Irish girls were delighted with the pile of Cadbury's.

Three

'Isn't he lovely!'

I watched him charming them, feeling pathetically, irrationally proud. The brisk-brusque nurse watched him too, arms folded, saying nothing until he left: 'So that's him?' And I wondered what I'd been saying when I was semi-conscious.

He took another day off work the following day, claiming to be at a conference in Liverpool, and returned to collect me. I felt a wrench leaving the other girls with whom I had formed such a bond, knowing we could never keep in touch.

The clinic made sure I was armed with contraceptive pills before I was discharged.

On the way home we stopped at a shabby pub for a silent drink, and I lay on the banquette, at eye level with the dust and debris in the upholstery, body aching, shocked and sad, but mostly relieved, enormously relieved, because I would not have to face the catastrophe of telling my mother.

'Is she all right?' asked the barmaid, clearing glasses from the next table.

'She's got an upset stomach,' my boss replied, smiling at her. 'Maybe bring her a port and brandy.'

She put the port and brandy on the table in a bulbous, womb-shaped glass, just above my eye level, where it glowed a deep blood red.

The clinic gave me green discharge papers, which I folded tight and kept at the back of my bedside drawer because I could not throw them away. A friend said, 'Get rid of them!' and made me promise to do so, but I couldn't. I took them out occasionally and studied the mainly indecipherable details scrawled by hand, 'Weeks Gestation: 9...'; it seemed important that I keep some evidence that this thing had happened.

For everyone else it was over, but not for me. As the relief faded, I was left with a sense of loss and grief. I never regretted the decision I made – in the end there had been no option – but I deeply regretted that the decision had had to be taken at all.

I felt a sadness and loneliness that I could not verbalise. I worked out when the baby would have been born and was aware of the date each year when it passed. I followed the fortunes of Cecil Parkinson's daughter, Flora, with intense interest.

For six years I occasionally talked to friends about what had happened, but then I decided to leave it behind – it would not be part of my story any more.

I hardly mentioned it again, but it was part of my story; it was always part of my story. Years after, when Cello asked me how long it took me to get over having the abortion, I told him it took twelve years, until I gave birth to Nina.

I had always wanted children, but I wanted them with a reliable man, and I was bad at finding reliable men. I was afraid that the longer it took to find one, the greater the chance of my not being able to get pregnant when I wanted to. Perhaps that would be payback, punishment for having had an abortion at all.

The biological clock is a real thing; I heard it ticking loud and insistent throughout my twenties.

When I was twenty-nine and had been going out with Cello for two years, I told him I wanted to get married and have a baby, and if he wasn't interested to let me know now and, no hard feelings, I loved him and everything, but if that wasn't what he wanted I'd find someone else.

He was two years younger than me and taken aback. 'Er, right, okay, yes, right…' A twenty-seven-year-old man can wait forever; a twenty-nine-year-old woman who wants more than one child, not as long.

We were married the following year.

We had a few days in New York after the wedding, with a

second 'proper' honeymoon planned shortly after to Sri Lanka, Thailand and Hong Kong. After returning from New York, I went to the doctor's for the Far East inoculations and as the nurse held the loaded needle to my arm she asked, 'You couldn't be pregnant, could you?' I said it was unlikely, but she put the needle down, saying she'd better play safe and do a test.

An hour or two later, back at my desk at work, I got a phone call from the nurse: 'Are you sitting down...?'

I phoned Cello and asked him to meet me at home, I had some news. I bought a bottle of champagne on the way.

I kept that receipt for years, too.

Despite being pregnant, I headed off to the Far East, even after the doctor said, '*Some* people wouldn't go.'

I was nauseous from the moment we sat down for dinner on the first night in Colombo and a waiter flambéed a steak at a neighbouring table, as my stomach wrenched and heaved.

The sickness got worse in Bangkok. I worked hard to ignore the stomach-churning all-day nausea, trying to enjoy the tuk-tuks, the crowds and the tropical rainfall and pretend the holiday had not been a terrible mistake.

On arrival in Hong Kong, I started bleeding and had to abandon our hotel and any pretence that this was still a holiday, as I retreated to a friend, John's, flat on Hong Kong Island, dry-heaving, not knowing if I'd lost the baby.

I lay on the sofa sipping cold water as Cello played Scrabble, drank beer and chatted with John on the sunny balcony. John brought me gifts of lightly cooked fish, bunches of flowers and, best of all, anti-nausea wristbands that allowed me to crawl off the sofa for the odd shower. John phoned his GP father for advice and was told that my continued sickness indicated the baby was likely to be alive but there was no way of knowing for a few weeks until it was visible on a scan.

One Body

Nowadays, when I hear a father-to-be say, 'We are pregnant', I remember my all-encompassing nausea, against the backdrop of fun on the balcony, and think nope, it is only the person with the dividing cells inside them who is pregnant. And when I hear people say, 'You're not ill, just pregnant,' I think, 'Define ill'.

After seven days, a doctor at a Hong Kong hospital gave me a 'Fit to Fly' certificate and British Airways flew me home, missing out the week on a Sri Lankan beach altogether. I lay across the extra seat they gave us, my head in Cello's lap fantasising about cold weather and plain Ryvita, scones and Granny Smiths.

Nina was born seven months later.

Two years later, I phoned for the results of my last pregnancy test using Cello's first mobile phone, as we stood in front of John Menzies on Princes Street, looking up at Edinburgh Castle. They were endless moments as I stood with fingers crossed listening to the receptionist shuffling papers and clunking the phone until she picked it up again: 'It's positive.'

That view of Princes Street Gardens, Castle Rock and the Edinburgh skyline still sends a joyful thrill right through me.

Four

At soon as my breast cancer was confirmed, I was told I must stop taking hormone replacement therapy (HRT). Lizzie, the breast care nurse, explained that my cancer was 'ER Positive', which meant it thrived on oestrogen and as a result the HRT was feeding the tumour.

Back home, I took my HRT tablets from the kitchen shelf and opened the bin but could not bring myself to throw them away, hiding them on the top of a kitchen cupboard instead. I could never take another, but I could not bear to let them go.

I had started taking HRT ten years before, aged forty-four, after going through an early menopause at forty-two. HRT had made me feel normal again. It had made me feel like 'me'. I had vowed that if any medic ever tried to take my HRT away from me, I would source it on the internet, go abroad, find the money to pay for it; I would beg, steal or borrow to get my hands on it. I would *never* stop taking it.

And now here I was being told I had already taken my last one. I had to go cold turkey. There was no alternative.

The sense of loss was enormous. When I went on HRT it took away the hot flushes, the anxiety and the brain fog that came with the early menopause. It had stopped the panic attacks and the palpitations that were interfering with my ability to look after my two primary school-aged children. It had also, I hoped, been protecting my bones because when I was forty, I was diagnosed with osteopenia – the bones in my arms and legs were weaker than normal.

It had been shocking to face the menopause at forty-two; wasn't the menopause for grandmothers?

My GP told me I was too young for the menopause. It took eighteen months and several visits before he did the blood tests and found that yes, indeed, I *had* reached an early menopause and he referred me to the Women's Health Clinic when I was forty-four.

It was not a subject I could talk about – it felt shameful, as though I had failed at something fundamental. I have always had a fear of failure, and here I was failing in a way I had not even realised I *could* fail. I managed to tell my husband I was starting HRT without once uttering the word 'menopause'.

I could not say it comfortably for years.

Staying young is so highly prized – looking young, acting young, feeling young are apparently all-important. The media implied that reaching menopause would make me invisible, useless, finished. It was a stigmatised subject, a slide towards as-good-as-being-dead. I tentatively asked a friend: who were menopausal women supposed to be invisible to? To which she replied, 'Oh, men don't want to have sex with them any more.'

My mother had not hit the menopause until she was fifty-five – not something she ever talked about, except for one remark: 'I thought it was never going to happen.' Daughters often follow their mothers in this regard, so being thirteen years earlier than my mother increased the shock.

I was due a period on the day my mother was buried. It never came. I dashed out of the house in my black trouser suit to meet the hearse containing her coffin as it pulled up outside the farmhouse, wondering why I had no stomach cramps. They never came either. Associating this ending of an era with the burial of my mother highlighted the sense of me ageing by an entire generation on that one single day.

Menopause was not something women in their early forties talked about. It seemed a far-off place and time for most of us;

indeed, my contemporaries were often still considering having babies. I felt young and fit and vigorous. To discover I had hit the menopause at forty-two was like someone pressing the fast-forward button.

Menopause is a taboo subject, but *early* menopause is an especially lonely place. It is only now, when I talk about it openly, more than ten years later, that I find other women saying, 'That happened to me too.'

The day I went to the Women's Health Clinic to discuss my early menopause I felt awkward in the waiting room. I avoided eye contact with everyone. I did not want to be there.

I was seen by a grey-haired woman doctor whose first question was: 'Do you want any more children?' No. 'Well, we don't need to worry about that then,' she said, putting aside some leaflets.

She told me in no uncertain terms that taking HRT at my age was 'no different from a diabetic taking insulin'. She said she would expect my body to be producing these hormones still; but as it wasn't, it made sense to take them in tablet form.

I was aware of the research linking HRT to breast cancer, but I knew this research was controversial. I found this experienced, confident, no-nonsense doctor very reassuring. She was emphatic about the benefits of HRT. There was something about her wiry hair and scrubbed face that made her words seem truer, more trustworthy.

She was also telling me what I wanted to hear. It was a relief to be told I could take a tablet to stop the symptoms of the menopause and protect my osteopenic bones from osteoporosis.

But on that day, the thought of breast cancer was nowhere. Not mentioned. I left the clinic with my first box of HRT and walked along the elegant terrace of Georgian houses knowing that an era in my life had passed. I had been struggling on my own with the early menopause for two years by then and here I was officially declared post-menopausal. My reproducing days were over – at an age when a lot of men and some women had not even started.

I did not miss having painful periods, but it was still a mental shift to put that stage of life behind me. Indeed, it was dizzying.

The menopause felt like a catastrophic end to something, not the beginning of something else. I was a dusty, decrepit Miss Haversham wanting to put the clock back. I felt useless, diminished, speeding away from my still-fertile contemporaries. It was not growing old itself I feared – it is the lucky ones who get to be old – but I wanted to age at the same rate as everyone else. I didn't want to be singled out.

In many ways, an early menopause foreshadowed the isolating experience of getting breast cancer ten years later.

My mother was secretive about her age, as though a woman's age was private because it was a liability. I have always made a point of being the opposite. I loathe the sniggering, patronising phrase 'a woman of a certain age'. I treat each birthday as yet another year of memories and experiences in the bank – years that no one can take away from you – but this plunging into early menopause *was* shaming.

I could not talk about it. I was silenced by this taboo subject; I have always found it hard to know when to keep quiet, when to talk, what to reveal and what to conceal, but on this subject my lips were sealed.

Fertility is such a huge part of a woman's life; so much time and energy spent dreading getting pregnant, trying to get pregnant, grieving the inability to get pregnant, getting pregnant, trying to stay pregnant, trying not to stay pregnant. But by my early forties that chapter was closed.

I decided to celebrate rather than cry, even if it would be a private celebration with only me there. At the end of the Women's Health Clinic's Georgian terrace was a vintage jewellery shop.

Four

I had browsed in it before, fascinated by the stories that lurked and swirled among the brooches, the necklaces, the beads and the clip-on earrings. By all of the women who had worn them before.

I have always loved jewellery. As a five-year-old, I sidled to the front of the primary school class during hymn practice to stroke the teacher's rings as she played 'All Things Bright and Beautiful' on the upright piano.

Walking past that day, I decided that jewellery would be my celebration and my consolation. I went in and examined the displays in the glass cases and saw a string of jade beads with a dangling green Buddha. The assistant was stylish in a black vintage dress and sparkling brooch and looked as though she could be placed back in one of her own display cases at the end of the day. She explained that the beads were not jade but 'Peking glass', a substance developed in China to resemble jade – but which was cheaper and easier to work.

They were not in fact cheap; they were expensive, but I wanted to treat myself kindly and at least pretend to celebrate.

I bought them and headed home on the bus, the HRT in my bag that I hoped would make me feel better, and the beads dangling around my neck that I clutched for comfort and for luck; not jade but faux jade. Not stone but glass. Not what they seemed.

I felt relief that there was a solution to my symptoms, but I also felt *different*; I had jumped a decade overnight and left my contemporaries behind. I was facing something they were not. I was alone, with something else to be ashamed of, something else to stay silent about.

Shame seems to me to be a constant companion when you live in a woman's body.

Five

My mother died of non-Hodgkin's lymphoma in 2006 after a debilitating and painful experience of chemotherapy treatment that lasted six years. She blamed her cancer on a mammogram that went wrong. I have asked medical friends over the years and been assured that my mother's fears cannot have been grounded in fact.

But she believed it.

She told the story many times of how she was first on the mammogram machine that morning, and how the machine made a loud bang, how the nurse appeared to panic and had to reset the machine and how she got my mother to redo the mammogram. Within days my mother's skin had begun to burn and flake around her breast and her back. Pretty soon she had open weeping sores on her raw torso. She showed them to me, lifting her blouse to reveal her red, flaking back, baffled and upset and outraged. She had never had skin trouble before. She went to the doctor's, who gave her skin cream. When she explained about the mammogram, they gave her antidepressants. She brought them home and, in a fury, flushed them down the toilet.

She refused to return to the GP even though she started suffering from stomach problems, restless leg syndrome and headaches. Eventually, after several years, by which time she could eat nothing but the powdered meal replacement Complan, she was forced back to the doctors where she eventually discovered she had non-Hodgkin's lymphoma.

She wrote to the Health Service Ombudsman to explain what had happened at the mammogram but was told she had left it too late to make a complaint.

Women in Scotland are offered mammograms every three years from the age of fifty, but after my mother's experience I swore I would never set foot in a mammogram clinic.

My fiftieth birthday came and went, and no invitation arrived. I was glad. I did not chase it up. A few months later I spotted what looked like a shipping container marked *Scottish Breast Screening Programme Mobile Screening Unit* parked beside the local Tesco. It was overlooking a Kwik Fit, not far from Tesco's back door, where the staff in their fleeces hung out to smoke. 'How horrible,' I thought gazing at it, from the far side of the car park, beyond the trollies, 'how sordid. I'm never going there.'

Then a friend's wife went and was diagnosed with breast cancer. The 'horrible' mobile unit had saved her life.

So, when my invitation did arrive, I plucked up the courage and went for my first mammogram in 2014, aged fifty-one.

The experience was not the trauma I had expected. I was asked to strip to the waist by a female mammographer and each breast was separately squashed between two plates and X-rayed for a few seconds. It felt primitive and a little brutal, but for me it was uncomfortable rather than painful – unlike smear tests, which are supposed to be pain-free, but I find agonising.

Shortly afterwards I received the standard letter (the *thin* letter – you always want a *thin* letter in response to medical tests). *I am pleased to tell you that your recent breast X-ray examination was satisfactory and showed no evidence of cancer.* Phew. No bangs. No panicked nurse. No erupting skin. No cancer.

But four years later in 2018, when my next invitation arrived for a mammogram, my fears had returned. Did I want to go again?

Many women are unsure, so the invitation comes with a leaflet – breast cancer is *built* from leaflets – listing potential concerns such as: the mammogram may miss a cancer; the mammogram may lead to a diagnosis of non-invasive cancer that would have done you no harm; very rarely, the X-rays may cause breast cancer; and the mammogram may cause anxiety and discomfort.

Most women, of course, are not terrified by their mother's belief that they were killed by a mammogram and nowhere in the leaflet does it suggest that you should be concerned that the mammogram machine may explode and cause non-Hodgkin's lymphoma.

What advice would my mother have given me if she were still alive?

I know she never went for another mammogram and I wondered if her legacy was to keep me safe from mammograms?

The leaflet said breast cancer was the most common cancer in women and added: *For every 400 women screened regularly for 10 years, one less woman will die from breast cancer.*

Was that 'one less woman' me? Was I the one to be saved?

I searched for reasons not to go and, as usual, when in doubt, I searched for answers from writers.

Sitting in bed one night, Cello quoted from a book he was reading, written by the scientist Sue Black: '…for myself, I cannot see the point in going to a doctor so that they can look for something that might be wrong when there is no indication right now of any problem'. Apparently, Sue Black's grandmother always warned her to stay away from hospitals, and she goes on, 'I don't want my life to be hampered by the constraints of a diagnosis or prognosis, to be defined by an illness or to become a medical statistic.'

I thought of my mother's mammogram and my ninety-two-year-old father's lifelong aversion to doctors, and I nodded sagely. Yes, that made sense. My determination to avoid the mammogram strengthened.

I then discovered an article by the writer Barbara Ehrenreich, entitled: 'Why I'm giving up on primary care'. Ehrenreich described the upset of having a 'false-positive' from a mammogram, which made her so stressed she got a 'distracted driving' ticket, before being told by her doctor that no treatment was necessary. She decided she was 'old enough to die' and 'old enough not to incur any more suffering, annoyance or boredom in the pursuit of a longer life'. She would go for no more mammograms, nor screening of any sort. She was 'no longer interested in looking for problems that remain undetectable to me'.

I admired her decisiveness when she said, 'Being old enough to die is an achievement, not a defeat, and the freedom it brings is worth celebrating.'

I Googled her and discovered she was seventy-seven years old – twenty-three years older than me – which made me realise with clarity that I wanted to live long enough to be a fearless old lady like Barbara Ehrenreich.

So, in June 2018 I went for my second mammogram.

I had moved and it was no longer in the mobile unit at Tesco, but in an actual clinic. I headed off on the bus, unsure where it was. After 20 minutes I asked the bus driver, 'Where is...' I rooted in my handbag for the appointment letter, 'er...'

'The breast place?' he asked cheerfully. He must have been used to lost middle-aged women wearing easy-to-slip-on-and-slip-off tops asking for directions. 'It's that,' he said, pointing to an ugly building at the end of a row of tenements.

I thanked him, jumped off the bus and ran across the road, wanting to get this over so I could forget about mammograms and breast cancer for another three years.

Now, two months later, normal life had ended as jarringly as if my sledge had hit a grassy patch and thrown me off.

Breast cancer was confirmed, but I was still facing uncertainty until after the lumpectomy and the lymph nodes had been examined. Trying to picture the next few months was like looking through a glass darkly. What treatment would I need besides surgery? How ill would it make me? Would I lose my hair? Would I be able to work? Was I in effect jumping off the world for a while? And if so, did 'jumping off the world' sound, in some odd way, like a relief?

I Googled 'jumping off the world' and up popped a video about BASE jumping. Well, if nothing else, I knew I wouldn't be doing that.

I sat back at my desk in my Edinburgh flat listening to the usual city centre noises, muted from being three storeys up: the drilling of road works, the droning of traffic and crashing of glass recycling, the blaring of car horns and snatches of car radio, the shouts of the homeless man, Stevie, who berates the world when he isn't slumped under his blanket.

Life was carrying on.

I gazed down on the pedestrians, some marching, some strolling, dodging in and out of shops and restaurants, crossing the street, the odd one dragging a wheelie case, and I wondered which of them had also hit a grassy patch; which of these people apparently going about their daily business were actually as stunned as me?

On the evening of the diagnosis, I read one of my short stories at the launch of a literary magazine in a local book shop. I did not mention cancer. I spent the evening back in that disconcerting parallel world pretending everything was normal.

The story had some funny lines and people laughed, which felt good but unreal. I was a fake, pretending.

But how is someone who has been diagnosed with cancer that day supposed to act?

The day after the diagnosis, I visited my GP's surgery for blood tests to ensure I was fit for the operation. The nurse took three phials of blood, and as she filled in the forms, she said, 'You're lucky. If you are going to get any cancer, let it be breast cancer.' She tapped away on her keyboard. 'They've spent such a lot on research.' I found myself nodding, despite being taken aback to be told I was lucky.

But as I walked home the thought struck me: just because I had breast cancer, it did not mean that in the future I wouldn't get another kind of cancer – a less well-funded, less-understood cancer. I had an urge to run back to the surgery to point out that fate does not decree everybody only has one once-in-a-lifetime cancer. That perhaps I was not 'lucky' after all.

My GP gave me a sheet entitled *Living with and beyond cancer – identifying your concerns*. On it were six categories of 'concerns': there were twenty-three 'physical concerns', ranging from constipation to nightmares to sexuality; there were nine 'practical concerns', including work, money and travel insurance; three 'family concerns' about partners or children; nine 'emotional concerns', such as anger, guilt and loneliness; three 'spiritual concerns', including loss of faith and loss of purpose in life; and eight 'lifestyle needs', including diet and exercise.

The list of potential problems was vast, too big to face. I shoved the sheet in my handbag and left it there for months.

It is difficult to absorb information after a cancer diagnosis. I wanted to talk, but appointments were short, doctors were busy, questions were tricky – you didn't know what you didn't know. Even if you wrote down your questions, they seemed pointless or inconsequential once you were in the doctor's office. Information was often given in leaflets that seemed incomprehensible and inaccessible at first but were at least still there when the time was right.

I still could not tell everyone because Lara was in the USA for another two weeks. I had a strong desire to articulate it, though. I told my sister over the phone: it was the first time I had spoken the words out loud. *I have breast cancer.* They sounded bizarre coming from my mouth and were met with a ringing silence, then, 'I don't know what to say.'

I had blurted it out because she wanted me to commit to a visit involving a four-hour journey down south. I was reluctant to plan anything until I knew more about my situation, so I said, 'I have breast cancer.' The words formed a bubble in front of me and burst in my face. As they echoed in my head, I felt horror, but also relief – because, surely, no one could expect anything from me now.

Did this diagnosis come with a Get Out of Jail Free card? Would it give me the strength to be honest at last? Would it give me permission to say 'no' when I needed to? Would it help me work out what I really wanted?

Another friend told me I was lucky. She was going through treatment for breast cancer herself and believed, like the nurse, that breast cancer was better funded than most cancers. I found myself agreeing without knowing if it was true or not. I realised that although I was going to be sensitive about what people said to me regarding cancer, if someone had had cancer themselves, that gave them licence to say whatever they liked about it, absolute carte blanche, no matter how much I disagreed with them.

I confided in a friend who had been treated recently for cervical cancer. She sounded sad and angry when she told me people had crossed the street to avoid her because they found gynaecological cancers 'so embarrassing'. In that moment I felt, if not lucky, then relieved that I had cancer of the breast, a 'non-embarrassing' cancer nowadays, a sanitised, pink beribboned, commodified cancer. It underlined for me yet again how shamed women are made to feel about their bodies.

The previous fifteen years had been difficult: my mother's lingering death from cancer twelve years ago, my early menopause, my younger sister's struggle with mental ill health and her suicide four years ago, trying to support a grieving elderly parent, raising two children – one of them autistic – while my husband and I worked as self-employed freelance writers right through the 2008 crash. There had been no wriggle room, never a moment to take stock.

It hit me that perversely this diagnosis might not be all bad.

Maybe this was what I had meant by the sensation of 'jumping off the world' – a letting go of certain obligations, a letting myself off the hook. I could not openly admit this; how bad was I at saying 'no' if it took cancer to improve things?

Searching for comfort and answers, I stumbled upon a claim that the Chinese word for 'crisis' was made up of two characters: 'danger' and 'opportunity'.

Was this true? Apparently, the phrase *Chinese word for crisis* has its own Wikipedia page; President Kennedy had mentioned the phrase in campaign speeches. However, 'American linguist Benjamin Zimmer' poured cold water on the 'danger and opportunity' definition, describing it as 'wishful thinking'.

I decided to disregard American linguist Benjamin Zimmer and wrote in my notebook:

Crisis = Danger + Opportunity.

Six

My uncle Dennis used to call make-up 'war paint' to put us off wearing it. *I see you've getten your war paint on again!* It didn't work. Nothing could put us off wanting to paint our faces, not even being compared to the baddies in the Westerns – characters who in the seventies were depicted as war-whooping savages. I would have been even keener if I had known Native American warriors painted their faces as a protective talisman, to help them gain health, strength and courage.

My first lipstick, bought from Boots in Lancaster when I was twelve, was orange, in a silver case. It was called 'Dancing' by Maybelline. My second was strawberry-flavoured roll-on lip gloss, which was not unlike applying a layer of jam. I first started smearing creams onto my face when my big sister introduced me to Astral – a thick white lotion in a blue pot – when I was barely out of primary school.

Over the years I enjoyed buying lotions and potions, even after a friend who worked for a big pharmaceutical company told me, 'If any of it actually worked, you'd have to get it on prescription.'

The power of make-up drove me to Harvey Nichols the day after diagnosis to buy red lipstick.

Suddenly I *needed* red lipstick.

I hovered near the make-up counters, self-conscious, performing the part of a relaxed shopper – make-up had become more complicated in the past few years and certainly since the days of 'Dancing' lipstick and *Jackie* magazine. There had been many years when my children were young when I hardly wore make-up at all.

A young woman attendant asked if I needed help. I told her I needed red lipstick. I had never worn red lipstick and was not sure I *could* wear red lipstick, but today I needed it. Red lipstick signalled defiance, strength and purpose. In the circumstances, pinks, plums, browns and nudes did not cut it.

I once read about the liberation of Bergen-Belsen death camp and how when a consignment of lipsticks arrived, the young British soldiers were amazed at the enormous morale boost it provided to the dehumanised, starving women, who wandered the camp dressed in rags and red lipstick, even to the point, the soldiers believed, of making the difference between life and death.

I did not mention the Holocaust to the assistant in Harvey Nicks.

She gave my face a searching look and said she knew the exact shade. I perched on a bar stool beside the make-up counter as she bustled around, returning with a lipstick called 'Ruby Woo, a retro matte vivid blue-red'. She drew a bold line around my lips then coloured them in with a cotton bud covered in Ruby Woo. I had images of Ronald McDonald selling burgers.

'Do I look like a clown?'

She assured me I did not and passed me a mirror. This lipstick would require confidence – real or faked – and I needed that.

I blurted out, 'I have breast cancer.'

I needed to practise the words, to repeat them, because I could not accept them.

She started backwards and said she was sorry, then declared she would make up my face to match the red lipstick. She produced a bundle of accessories like a workie's tool set and applied bronzer and highlighter with big fluffy brushes, concentrating hard, dabbing and sweeping like an Old Master at a canvas. I focused on her swinging hoop earrings to avoid awkward eye contact as she painted my eyelids, shaped my eyebrows and applied mascara until, again, she handed me the mirror.

I looked different. No longer terrified, cowed or haunted. I looked strong, and definitely not invisible. I did not look like a woman who had just discovered she had breast cancer (whatever that woman looks like).

I bought the lot for £114.59. For a bag of confidence – real or faked – that seemed reasonable.

Thirty-five years ago my grandma Mary died of ovarian cancer, but I only recently found a little red recipe book that must have been hers among my other recipe books in a kitchen drawer. There were eight sections, including Entrees, Meat, Game & Poultry, Jellies & Ices, but the only section with recipes written in her handwriting, the same handwriting I recognised from numerous birthday cards (*Fondest Love, Grandma x*), were in the Cakes & Pastries section: Doris's Ginger Beer, Egg Flip, Slab Cake, Parkin, Lunch Cake, Thora Hird's Aunty Wynn's Cake. The rest of the book was empty except for one handwritten entry in 'Soups':

Beauty Cream

1oz White Wax, 5oz Almond Oil, 4oz Rose Water, a few drops of Scent, 1oz of Spermaceti…

I blink. Yes, '1oz of Spermaceti'. I Googled and discovered Spermaceti was 'a waxy substance found in the head cavities of the Sperm Whale … used chiefly in ointments and cosmetic creams…'.

The recipe continued:

Warm the Wax and Spermaceti in a pan, keep stirring, add the Almond Oil and Rose Water, add the Scent last, when cool. Apply for beauty.

This recipe must have been written by Grandma in the 1960s when she was in her fifties – my age now. At the time, she resembled the Queen Mother, with a beatific smile. I remember her getting her grey-white hair done every Friday by Aunty Dorothy, using setting lotion and rows of little pink curlers and a vicious sharp-ended comb in the farmhouse kitchen. I remember her wearing a fur coat with glittery peacock and poodle brooches and a hat coated with feathers for evensong, and I remember her sequined frocks for Ladies Evenings and the Farmers Ball. I remember her gold necklaces and her many-mirrored dressing table, her bottles of cologne and her silk scarves knotted under her chin like the Queen, but I don't remember her wearing make-up or putting anything on her face at all.

Make-up was treated with suspicion; it had the power to change you – probably into someone who was 'no better than they ought to be'. *Wipe that muck off yer face*, Grandad would say to us. I do not remember Grandma cooking up a pan of Beauty Cream on her stove, stirring it like a spell, but I wish I did.

I told my twenty-three-year-old daughter Nina as soon as the cancer was confirmed.

I said I had a tumour, which was *very* small and would be removed *very* soon. I found myself avoiding the word 'cancer', like the doctors had. I explained I would have radiotherapy and possibly chemotherapy. I saw the look of shock and fear cloud her face and I carried on talking to get us past the moment.

Sometimes I am not good at allowing quietness to settle because I am frightened of what it will reveal.

I did the entire spiel hovering near her bedroom door. I did not even sit down, in the mistaken belief that keeping it short would minimise the whole thing. 'Okay?' I said, with a forced smile, 'so nothing to worry about then', while rubbing my hands and bobbing about for a second, before edging to the door and being propelled out of the bedroom by my own sigh of relief.

I knew I had done it wrong, but what was the right way to tell your daughter you have breast cancer?

Little was said about it in the following days. Cancer was not mentioned over the dinner table. Within days Nina had begun to suffer from a severe, and apparently chronic, anxiety-related gut problem.

Weeks later I asked her how she felt on hearing the news and she said, 'I knew if you died it was my neck on the chopping block next. I felt death swirling around me.'

Two weeks later, Lara arrived home from America. She was excited and wanted to head straight into the city for a cocktail. 'It's Happy Hour,' she said, 'let's celebrate!'

Finding the right moment was going to be hard.

We arrived at the bar ten minutes early, so went next door into a high-end travel agent specialising in long-haul holidays. It was light and airy, and everything was cream, a temple to luxury travel. Lara suggested we find a holiday to celebrate her twenty-first birthday in five months.

I could not picture life in five months. It was a blank. I didn't know if I would have the strength to climb the three flights of stairs to our flat in five months never mind fly to another country.

Cello avoided the charade and hovered by the window as Lara and I perched on cream leather sofas beside a cream orchid. I asked about direct flights from Edinburgh next January, but the assistant sensed my half-heartedness and lost interest. She wandered off, leaving us leafing through glossy brochures.

Back at the bar, we got our cocktails and I said, 'I've got some news.' I had the sensation of teetering on a wobbly diving board.

A look of dread flashed across Lara's face and she became guarded.

'Don't tell me if it's bad news,' she said.

She told me later I looked defeated at that point, but I ploughed on.

'They have found a tumour in my breast.'

Again, I emphasised how '*very* small' it was and how they had caught it '*very* early' and again I avoided the word 'cancer'. She studied me, trying to read between the lines. I waved my hand in the region of my armpit as if to indicate 'it's so far up it's almost not breast cancer *at all*'.

I was doing what annoyed me when others did it: minimising; trying to conceal the depth of my terror.

Lara looked from me to Cello and back. 'So, you've known something was wrong for four weeks?'

'Yes.' I had flashbacks to our pretend-happy FaceTime conversations.

Lara nodded. 'Well, I'm glad I wasn't here when you found out. I'm glad I'm finding out now you've got your heads round it.'

I sighed with relief. We had done the right thing.

Then I realised with a shock that she thought I had got my head round it, when nothing, absolutely nothing, could have been further from the truth.

Seven

Death has always fascinated me, and before this diagnosis I believed – *really* believed – it was a subject I could 'handle' and I was proud of that, to the point where I was disdainful of those who could not.

My grandad died when I was ten and we were taken to see him in his coffin, embalmed and waxy. He was laid out, swathed in a white satin shroud in a satin-lined oak coffin in the best sitting room of his farm. There was a yellow hue to his face. I realised at that moment that death was inert – something had vanished from Grandad – this state was far, far away from sleeping and I was fascinated.

After the funeral, my cousins and I were encouraged to pick flowers and take them to his grave. I enjoyed the snippets of stories in the graveyard, the names of the dead and the fragments of their lives: husbands buried fifty years after their wives, children buried before their parents, young men fatally wounded at Arras in 1917 and Normandy in 1944. 'Dearly beloved wife of...', 'Devoted husband of...' Graveyards were as much about the living as the dead. They were not frightening; they were fascinating places to go to on a day out.

Every year the pupils at my village primary went on a school trip – there were just enough of us in the school to fill a coach. Usually it was to Chester Zoo or Rufford Old Hall, but in 1971 we went to visit 'Little Black Sambo's Grave'. We set off on the twenty-mile journey to Sunderland Point, a village among the marshes on the wind-blown peninsula between the mouth of the River Lune and Morecambe Bay, clutching our Mother's Pride bread wrappers containing egg butties and Blue Ribands.

We were told that 'Little Black Sambo' was a slave boy who

died in 1736 when his ship was in port. The plaque on his grave read: *Here lies poor Samboo, a faithfull Negro who (attending his master from the West Indies) died on his arrival at Sunderland.*

Mrs Darlington told us it was very sad that this child had died of a broken heart due to homesickness, and the villagers were kind to bury him here overlooking the water so he could be as near as possible to his homeland.

She mentioned neither Lancaster's part in the international slave trade, nor the riches brought to the area as a result; there was no mention that the grave was in fact dug here as it was unconsecrated ground because the dead child not being a Christian could not be buried in the churchyard.

After gazing at the grave for a while, we wandered off for our egg butties, unfazed by this gothic day out.

Nowadays there is a plaque on the grave bearing the words of the hymn 'Amazing Grace', written by slave-trader-turned-clergyman John Newton.

Back in 1971 I thought 'Amazing Grace' was a person.

As an adult, I prided myself on my non-hysterical, level-headed approach to death. I did not use euphemisms: the dead were 'dead', they had not 'passed', 'passed away' or 'passed on'; they were not 'asleep', 'lost' or 'slumbering'; being buried was 'being buried', not 'being laid to rest' or 'going home'.

A favourite day out is still to visit a historic graveyard to browse among the moss-covered, worn-smooth angels and cherubs and the carved skulls and crossbones. The epitaphs are both poetry and drama: 'Here lies the dust of…', 'Till their ashes be mouldering…', 'Until the daybreak and the shadows flee away…'. In the Glasgow Necropolis, the epitaph to Corlinda Lee, 'The Queen of the Gypsies', reads: 'Wherever she pitched her tent she was loved and respected by all.'

I scoffed when I heard about someone who refused to eat

potatoes from her husband's allotment because it was on an ancient burial ground. 'She won't eat vegetables grown in bones,' said my mother-in-law. When Cello refused to view a property overlooking a cemetery, I rolled my eyes. What better neighbours than the dead? I admired a (healthy) friend's practicality when he booked and paid for his own funeral at the Co-op, opting for a shroud in blue.

My father, sisters and I sat with Mum as she died of cancer in 2006. Afterwards I visited her body in the mortuary several times; I spoke to her, I took her glasses and lipstick and put them in her handbag in the coffin.

I was proud I could be in the presence of death.

When, a few weeks after the funeral, my dad said my mother's grave had sunk, I went with him to the churchyard and helped him remove the turf and wheeled barrowloads of soil from the back of the churchyard to level off the grave, before kneeling on it to smooth it out and relay the turf.

I was convinced I could deal with the reality of death.

Four years after my mother died, I began a writing project called *Body Disposal for Beginners,* to investigate the ways we can dispose of our bodies and how to arrange my own hypothetical funeral.

I interviewed a man who had buried his son in the front garden and a woman who sold woodland burial plots. I enjoyed the macabre thrill of being close to death, of dancing with it.

I attended an anatomy class at Edinburgh University because donating my body to medical science was a possibility, plus I relished the idea of testing my nerve: could I face death calmly in the anatomy rooms?

I believed so.

As I approached the professor's office in the Medical School, I passed specimen cases of bent and twisted spinal columns labelled 'scoliosis of the lower spine' and realised that, despite my bravado, I was nervous.

The professor smiled from behind his desk. His office was small and cluttered and a skeleton in a straw hat grinned over his left shoulder.

He led me upstairs to the anatomy rooms, through a door barring entry to the public and forbidding photography. It was an enormous, light-filled space, overlooking an interior courtyard, where fifty first-year students donned white coats and plastic gloves.

There was a stink of formaldehyde.

Today they were studying the chest wall and the respiratory system.

On a table lay a body with the skin removed and tiny numbered flags sticking out of various muscles in the chest. The rest of the body was swathed in cream-coloured cloth.

I was disappointed the undergraduates were not going to dissect a complete, recognisably human body like in Rembrandt's *The Anatomy Lesson of Dr Nicolaes Tulp*, but instead would examine already-dissected pieces.

Students wandered between the workstations; one contained a stack of ribcages, another a dangling skeleton, and the next had four large, white plastic trays containing human torsos, with the ribs removed and the trachea and diaphragm exposed. The students carried workbooks with dotted lines to fill in when they had identified certain muscles and body parts. Most had a *Gray's Anatomy for Students* stuck under their arm. As they asked each other if they had got this or that muscle identified, they brought to mind those I-SPY spotters' guides that middle-class kids had in the 1970s. *I-SPY Cars, I-SPY on the Pavement, I-SPY on a Train Journey* – except these kids had graduated to *I-SPY Sinews* or *I-SPY the Nervous System*.

The professor had warned me that the face, the feet and the fingers were what retained a person's humanity. And so it seemed. The hands on the complete body rested on the white cloth and were the hands of a grandmother, hands that could just have put down a book or stirred a cup of tea.

My legs felt shaky, so I perched on a chair and feigned writing notes.

After the lesson, the professor asked if I had seen the university's Anatomical Museum upstairs.

'We've got Burke's skeleton up there.' He got the key out of a drawer. 'Do you want to have a look?' I grabbed my handbag.

On the top floor, the professor switched on the lights, which flickered into life, revealing specimen cases as far as the eye could see. He took me to Burke: a greying skeleton displayed beside his death mask, which showed the noose marks around his neck. A sign pegged to his ribcage said: *Irish (Male) The Skeleton of William Burke The Notorious Murderer hanged Edinburgh 28th January 1829.*

The professor left me to browse. I wandered alone, self-conscious in the enormous space, past other dangling skeletons, trying not to catch their eye.

The most arresting sight was the row upon row of death masks. Sir Walter Scott, Sir Isaac Newton, William Wordsworth and a gallery of other old men were there; eyes shut and mouths dragging slightly at the corners, as though death had caught them unawares and they were not best pleased about it.

The death masks reminded me of Grandad embalmed in his coffin all those years ago and I made a mental note to investigate having one made. Perhaps that would be an amusing vignette for my writing project.

When it became too oppressive being watched by the blind-eyed masks and dangling skeletons, I made my way to the door, flicked off the lights and walked out quick sharp.

The professor was in the hallway holding the stepladder for a workman who was vacuuming the skeletons of two Indian elephants. He gave me a friendly wave. I ran down the stone steps, across the echoing tiled hall and out into the fresh air of the university courtyard.

I was proud; I had done it; I had been calm in the presence of death.

I did not admit to myself, as I gulped the fresh air and headed under the university's carved portal, that I was practically running.

I was then aged forty-six and could tackle with enthusiasm a project organising my own funeral because I had never felt stronger. But contrary to my belief that I was cool with the idea of death, over the years I often found myself poring over articles on 'How to live to be a hundred' and mentally ticking off the boxes.

Don't Smoke. I could tick that box, having only smoked one day in my life – when I was fifteen at a friend's sixteenth birthday party where the table decorations were tubs of cigarettes. I smoked an entire tub, threw up in the dustbin and have never touched another.

Take Exercise. Through Jane Fonda's 'Going for the Burn' Lycra-clad aerobics of the eighties, gym memberships of the nineties, prenatal yoga, postnatal yoga, 'Tums, Bums & Thighs', Body Pump, Body Balance, tap dancing, the obsession with daily steps and now 'yoga for the over-fifties', vanity had kept me exercising.

Limit Alcohol Intake. Since being pregnant with Nina, yes, I could tick that box. True, in my teens and twenties I had been a regular binge drinker, starting with spirits sweetened with cordial aged fifteen, but that was a long time ago…

Eat a Healthy Diet & Maintain a Healthy Weight. Yep, brought up on home cooking, I believed I was lucky enough, rich enough, privileged enough, and had chopped enough salad, steamed enough veg and climbed on enough weighing scales to live two lifetimes.

I eagerly read interviews with centenarians who offered a smorgasbord of recommendations: drink three Miller High Life beers and a glass of whisky every day; drink tea; drink wine; avoid men; get a kiss every day; eat chocolate; mind your own business; keep connected; don't have children; eat raw eggs; eat lightly; eat sushi; eat cookies; eat cheese puffs; sleep for days on end; keep active; take naps; have faith; have fun; keep working; be happy; shovel snow; don't take any baloney; eat cake; grow your own food; eat junk food; drink Dr Pepper; be kind; do puzzles; dance the polka; crochet; eat bacon; keep calm; wear fancy underwear; soak in hot springs…

Part of me believed that if I did it right, if I followed enough rules and picked up enough tips and kept luck on my side, I could live forever. When I was forty, I told a friend, in all seriousness, 'I've decided to live to be a hundred' – as though all it took was for me to *decide*.

Before my cancer diagnosis, death was something that could be fended off and dodged forever. It was so far away as to be an impossibility.

George Saunders, when discussing the writing of *Lincoln in the Bardo*, said he loved 'thinking about death'. I nodded with recognition at that and said to myself, 'I thought that too, George. Oh yes, I thought that.'

I continued believing I loved thinking about death until a cancer diagnosis taught me that the difference between thinking about death as a healthy person and thinking about death as someone with cancer is as different as a roller-coaster ride from a motorway pile-up; one is fun, the other is potentially deadly.

I had been teasing myself with the idea of mortality, playing with it, and life had called my bluff.

One day, not long after diagnosis, I overheard a conversation:
'What about Old Mary, then?'
'Aye, she died.'
'Over a hundred, she was.'
I was on the periphery of the conversation; I didn't really know these people and had never heard of Old Mary, but one of the old men looked at me and said, 'It doesn't matter how long you get; you always want more.'
And I thought, 'Oh, I know.'

My mother died of cancer at seventy-four. My father had bone cancer in his shoulder at fifty-three and in his hip at fifty-seven; he had an operation to remove his shoulder blade, and radiotherapy followed by chemotherapy for his hip, but he still survives in his nineties.

A seventy-five-year-old great-uncle had got cancer at the same time as Dad. Apparently, there was nothing they could do for him except 'try to make him comfortable', but the doctors decided it was not in his interest to be told he was dying of cancer. This was the early 1980s, when the professionals held the power and the information, and patients could be deemed unable to cope with the truth; to be told you had cancer may be too much to bear, it may send you into a deathly spiral of despair. Why add to the patient's burden?

After he died, I asked my mother, 'Did he die peacefully? Did they make him comfortable?' She was sitting at the kitchen table drinking a cup of tea and replied, 'I don't know about that. They said at the end he was crying for his mother.'

My maternal grandad died of lung cancer at sixty-three

– having never smoked – and my maternal grandmother died of ovarian cancer at seventy-one.

I always said airily that I would die of cancer – I *knew* it – it was in the family, but I wasn't expecting it at fifty-four. The shock to my sense of self was devastating. Not only had I got cancer in my early fifties, but I was not cool about death at all; I was terrified and could barely function.

I was not the person I had believed myself to be. I was not leading the life I thought I would lead. The shock was total.

I read and re-read the letter from our insurance company: *Dear Ms Simpson, we are sorry to hear you are unwell and have to make a claim for critical illness…*

That letter was addressed to me. Me! 'Unwell and having to make a claim for critical illness.' Unbelievable.

Whatever I was doing, whether I was alone or in company, out and about or trying to sleep, the words 'I have cancer' were on repeat in my head. I have cancer. I have cancer. Always at the forefront of my mind. I have cancer.

Watching a TV drama with Cello, one of the characters, newly diagnosed with cancer, said, 'I'm not in the same place as you. I am on the other side. I want to be back where you are.'

And I nodded.

Why do we all think we are special, and it won't happen to us?

Or at least, why did I think I was special and it wouldn't happen to me?

Eight

A few days after arriving home, Lara suggested we go to a Britney concert in Blackpool. I thought having cancer would give me permission to say 'no', but I discovered it also compelled me to say 'yes' because gathering new experiences seemed of the utmost importance. Creating memories with my family was paramount.

Off we set, down the motorway caterwauling 'Oops! ... I did it again', with the car stereo on full blast. Lara wore her Britney 'Piece of Me' tour T-shirt as I tried not to think about the piece of me that was causing so much trouble.

Once in Blackpool we headed towards the Golden Mile. Golden it was not. On the streets behind the front, we felt we had travelled back in time.

'There's a Woolworths,' said Lara. 'They don't exist any more!'

Many of the people looked impoverished, thin and unhealthy. Twice we had to take detours to avoid ambulance crews dealing with patients flat out on the pavement, and not over-indulged revellers either, but elderly people, grey and collapsed.

'We look like the healthiest people here,' I said to Lara, 'and I've got cancer.'

I was gripped with the desire to 'make the most of it while you can'. We had afternoon tea in the art deco café with individual three-tier cake stands, we wandered under the bunting and the fairy lights down North Pier, drank pink gin, and browsed the stalls selling sparkly hats and Minnie Mouse headdresses: *Everything three quid!* We spent our last pound riding the carousel.

In the public toilet I saw scrawled on the cubicle wall: *Dear Freddie, my lovely husband, I'm sorry I couldn't be as slim as you*

*wanted me to be. I was curvy when we met, when we got married
and now. But now you say you have passed your survival time and
you don't need a woman like me any more, and your taste has changed.
Question is: I love you but with such an attitude are you worth a committed relationship? Remember I have travelled further than most to
walk by your side. And yes, this is a true story.*

I took a snap of it on my iPhone. How had Freddie 'passed his
survival time'? How had she 'travelled further than most'? What
did it mean? Why had she told her story in a toilet cubicle at the
end of North Pier? So many dramas playing out. Unseen. Below the
surface. So many people, living their stories and needing to share.

The concert was on the 'Comedy Carpet' between Blackpool
Tower and the sea front – an area where catchphrases, jokes and
song lyrics from the history of British comedy cover the ground. I
walked past 'Knickers, Knackers, Knockers!!!' And 'Ooh, I do feel
queer' as we joined Pitbull to sing 'Don't Stop the Party'.

Pit who?

Pitbull. You must have heard of Pitbull?!

Oh … right…

I could only see him through the screen of someone else's
iPhone held aloft in front of me.

We cheered Britney in her black and silver bondage gear, as she
gyrated under a neon sign saying 'Shameless', in the shadow of the
Tower, and when she yelled, 'How are you feeling, Birmingham?'
we frowned. *Did she say…?* I studied her up there, in the limelight,
knowing she was dealing with enormous health issues herself, but
still being Britney.

We smiled for selfies, even as we were herded by staff in head-
to-toe yellow hi-vis, jostled by the crowd, unable to get to the
toilets for hours, left standing for long periods with nothing to
entertain us except the lights flashing up and down Blackpool
Tower because the view of the sea was blocked by security

fencing. We were packed in, cheek by jowl, watched over by a police marksman on a neighbouring roof, as I had flashbacks to reports of the bomb at the Ariana Grande concert the year before. We stood our ground against drunken fans body-bumping us carrying fistfuls of overflowing plastic beer glasses above their heads, swaying in time to the music and singing with their eyes shut. And still we smiled for the selfies.

At one point a girl in the crowd turned around, looked me up and down, as I stood there in my grey *This Too Shall Pass* sweat-shirt with my exhausted ashen face, and she raised an eyebrow to Lara: 'Your mum dresses well.' Lara looked daggers at her, and I wanted to say, 'I've got CANCER! Bet you feel shit now!'

I used to take comfort from the phrase 'This too shall pass' and toyed with getting it tattooed on my arm. Now I am glad I didn't as I don't like to imagine the mortician's raised eyebrow, seeing me on the slab with that inked on my skin; because, yes, all things pass, but some things kill us in the passing.

After the concert we headed back to the hotel, worn out, no money left for a non-existent taxi. We were unable to find an open restaurant or a late-night shop able to take my bank card and as we stood among the tins of soup and packets of biscuits wondering what we could buy with our remaining coppers, we were gifted two bags of crisps by a sympathetic shopkeeper.

But it didn't matter that we were exhausted and hungry, with aching feet. What mattered was that we had created lots of memories and stocked them in the memory bank.

It had been worth it.

I had planned to keep the news quiet until we came back from the Italian wedding, but with a week to go I was done with keeping quiet. After weeks of whispering it to selected people, I needed to speak about it openly.

I phoned an elderly aunt.

'*Everybody* seems to have cancer now,' she said, with an air of disappointment and exasperation, as though she was considering writing a letter of complaint.

'I didn't want you to find out on Facebook,' I said.

'Oh, you don't want to be putting it on there,' she said.

But I did.

Messages of support flooded in. People sent ornaments and cards with pink ribbons on them. I was baffled until I realised it was the symbol for breast cancer and it was *everywhere*. How had I missed it?

As a child I adored pink. I coveted my doll's pink satin dress, wishing I could squeeze into it; I longed for my cousin's dressing table with its skirt of pink roses, and yet another cousin's pink pinafore. I wanted to be pink. Now I found myself in a world of pink: pink leaflets, pink cards, pink posters. If it was breast cancer, it was pink.

I no longer wanted to be pink, but it was too late.

People sent me angels: a ceramic angel, a jade angel, a crystal angel, a 'handmade guardian angel to look over you'. I was touched, even though I did not believe in the power of angels until one fell off a shelf, shattering its wing, and I was struck through with dread.

It was a relief to be done with the secret. Now I was a member of a new club, a sisterhood, the Breast Cancer Survivors' Club. Messages arrived: 'I'm a survivor too if you need to talk...', 'I've been there, I'm thinking of you...', 'If there's anything I can do...', 'My sister...', 'My mother...', 'My grandmother...'

Some people on social media included 'cancer survivor' in their bios: 'Knitter, yogi, breast cancer survivor.' 'Mother of five, breast cancer survivor.' 'Architect, engineer, breast cancer survivor.' I was grateful for their generosity in sharing this information because it made me feel less alone, but I wondered, when do you become a breast cancer survivor? How long do you have to survive to be a survivor?

As with most cancer questions, I Googled it. The answer seemed to be: it depends. One writer suggested that if you have been diagnosed with breast cancer then you are already a survivor: 'A person is a survivor on the day of diagnosis and for the rest of their lives.'

Another writer said that if I wanted to mark my 'cancerversary', the best date for describing myself as a survivor may be the day I completed my hospital-based treatment – the surgery and chemo and/or radiation. I doubted I would *ever* want to use the term 'cancerversary', but by that reckoning I had a long way to go before becoming a 'survivor'.

Shortly after spotting the 'breast cancer survivor' tag in one twitter bio, I noticed the owner had removed the words. She explained she got rid of the tag because, although it was true, it was not all she was. I replied, 'Thanks for having it there. It made me feel less alone.'

In chatrooms, some people named their cancer: 'I hope Beryl is gone now.' Others gave it a name that they believed helped them to 'fight' it, for example, 'Nancy' – short for malignancy – or a name that expressed anger or frustration, 'Lucifer' or 'Pita' – the latter standing for Pain in the Arse.

I did not name my cancer. It felt like part of *me* – which of course it was – my own flesh and blood. Weirdly, I felt sorry for the cells in my body that were getting it so wrong: mutating and putting so much effort into dividing away like mad, and yet, with luck, all of their effort would come to nothing. I almost felt protective of them. Almost.

Even though cancer had been a constant in my life since I was a ten-year-old child, I did not know what cancer *was* until I got it myself.

With Dad's cancer, I knew he had a 'lump' in his shoulder blade that had to be removed, and four years later another lump in his hip bone. Other than that: nothing. I did not wonder what the lumps were, or how cancer had formed such lumps.

Was this because I *thought* I knew what it was, so I didn't have to find out? Was it because I was too frightened to find out? Or was it because I trusted the doctors to tell us what we needed to know *if* we needed to know it?

But it was different now the cancer was in my own body. Now I *needed* to know as much as I could. I became obsessed with finding out.

I started in the way I always have, with the *Oxford Paperback Dictionary*, a book that has lived by my bedside since I was a teenager. I read it avidly then, although I don't remember ever looking up 'cancer'. The dictionary told me cancer was: *1. A tumour, especially a malignant one. 2. A disease in which malignant growths form. 3. Something evil that spreads destructively. 4. Cancer, a sign of the zodiac, the Crab.*

I flipped 300-odd pages to 'malignant'. In pre-internet days this was how I fell down the information rabbit hole, zigzagging from definition to definition. 'Malignant' according to this dictionary was: *1. (of a tumour) growing uncontrollably. 2. Feeling or showing great ill will.*

So, cancer was a tumour growing uncontrollably.

Or cancer was a disease in which uncontrollable growths form.

Or cancer was something evil spreading destructively.

Or cancer was a tumour showing great ill will.

Or Cancer was a star sign.

Or Cancer was a crab.

In fact, the disease is known as 'cancer' because the projections from the central tumour physically resemble a crab.

I was always glad I was a Scorpio.

I went to the bookshop. Did they have a cancer section? No, but they had a foot and a half of shelf marked 'Health and Well-being'. I came away with a memoir of Lyme disease and a celebrity cancer diary.

I went to the library. Did *they* have a cancer section? No, but they led me to the 'Family' shelves and there among the Depression and the Infidelity, the Child Rearing and the Sleep Hygiene, I found a steady trickle of cancer stories.

Desperate to know what I was in for, I dived in. From *Cancer: The Beginners Guide* to the Pulitzer Prize-winning *The Emperor of All Maladies: A Biography of Cancer*, I read about cancer as though my life depended upon it.

I trawled the internet searching for information to help prepare me for treatment. I was frightened of the long-term effects of radiotherapy – after all, radiation causes, as well as treats, cancer. I read that the therapeutic radiotherapy machines use much higher voltage than ordinary diagnostic X-ray machines – they are 1,000 times more powerful, so the X-rays penetrate deeper and cause more damage than ordinary X-rays.

I found the story of a woman who chose to have a full mastectomy – complete removal of the breast – rather than a lumpectomy, to avoid the need for radiotherapy. I told one or two people about this and they kept bringing it up: have you asked about a full mastectomy? Perhaps you'd be better off with a full mastectomy?

I regretted ever mentioning it and felt shaken: first, because I was too frightened to ask the question in case the answer was, yes, a full mastectomy is a good idea; and secondly, I didn't want to bother the medics. *Oh, no, someone else has been consulting Dr Google!*

Eventually I agreed to phone the breast care nurses at the Breast Unit and ask their advice. I phoned the number, hyperventilating with nerves, to be met by an answerphone: *You have phoned the line for the breast care nurses. Please leave your details and a brief summary of your query.*

I found it impossible to form the words that would constitute a 'brief summary' of whether I should have my breast amputated or not. I hesitated, I licked my lips, my mouth opened and closed wordlessly, then I slammed the phone down.

That night I had a dream that my breast was gone, that one side was completely flat. I woke up cold with dread, knowing I would go for the lumpectomy and radiation without asking any more questions.

Nine

Getting information about my body has never been easy, and knowing myself physically and mentally, and being able to talk about it, has been a long haul.

As a child on the farm, we witnessed cows calving, pigs farrowing and cats kittening as well as being familiar with the work of the AI – the artificial inseminator – and yet we were sent out of the way when Uncle Dennis's sows visited our boar. Presumably, this was to avoid awkward questions, but as a child I was annoyed: what could *possibly* be happening that I was not allowed to watch?

It was unsettling having something unknown and unspoken, both sniggeringly funny to my older cousins, yet at the same time embarrassing and shameful – and not just when the sows came. Why did an aunt laugh when I mentioned that another aunt and uncle were getting twin beds? Why did my mother laugh when I asked how God knew you were married before he gave you babies? How did I know, aged seven, to struggle and run when an elderly uncle said, 'Let's kiss like lovers do'?

Knowledge came in fits and starts. A girl in the village let it be known she had information; it was from a Ladybird book so it must be right, but I was deemed too young to be told by the other children. By the time the details filtered through, I was informed: the man's snake goes into the lady's grass', so I wasn't a lot nearer. I ran this information past my big sister, who laughed, 'Snake?! Grass?! That's not what they say at *my* school.'

One day, before I knew anything of periods or sanitary protection, I discovered an intriguing strappy white belt hanging in the bathroom and put it on over my trousers and danced into the kitchen in it. My mother and big sister were horrified: 'Put that back!' I withdrew, embarrassed and puzzled, unaware I had been disco-dancing in a device known as a sanitary belt – an elastic belt with metal clips used to hold a bulky sanitary pad in place until the early seventies – but knowing I had committed a shaming error. The incident was never mentioned again.

Puberty happened before I knew it, without preparation or warning – my body transforming before my startled eyes, like one of the werewolves in *American Werewolf in London*.

When the bleeding began, I forced myself to go to sleep, hoping it would have stopped by morning.

Nappy-like pads became part of life (thankfully now with modern adhesive strips rather than primitive belts, although it would be another few years until they were 'now with wings!'), but they still felt *enormous* and made you feel self-conscious all day. Despite the adverts showing laughing women horse-riding in white trousers while on a period, bleeding once a month felt like a severe restriction.

Fear and shame were the overriding emotions. The fear of being caught without protection, the fear of leaking – glancing back at the chair you had left in case it was smeared with blood, checking the back of your skirt – the fear of the pad coming adrift, the fear of smelling like blood, the dread of the cramps and the pains, the fear of the pad being visible through PE shorts, the fear of anyone *knowing*. Even among a group of close girlfriends at school, no one mentioned periods.

There was the ever-present dread that your period would coincide with sleepovers, school trips, long journeys or anything else that would make changing and disposing of sanitary protection even more difficult.

But apparently not all girls were as inhibited. When a 'girls only' meeting was called by the female deputy head before an upcoming school trip at high school, I saw one thirteen-year-old girl mouth to another, 'It'll be about ower monthlies!' I was astounded that not only did this girl have a word to use, but that she dared to use it.

Visiting a friend, I was surprised but impressed to see boxes of Tampax left out in the bathroom, willy-nilly, *as though they just didn't care.* How sophisticated, I thought, putting it down to them being a houseful of intellectuals; working at Lancaster University was clearly another world.

Adverts for sanitary products emphasised 'discretion', but it felt like shameful secrecy to me. Pads started to come in boxes of individually wrapped items in plain wrapping for additional 'discretion' in your bag.

I would remove the adhesive strip from a pad while sitting on the loo at school, holding my breath, so as not to make any noise in the toilet cubicle. Cubicles were not fitted with disposal bins for used sanitary towels, and we were given dire warnings about the state of the school plumbing and instructed to use the communal clanking metal bin beside the handbasins. To emerge from the toilet cubicle with a sanitary towel to dispose of would have been a humiliation, so I wrapped my used pads in toilet paper, hid them at the bottom of my school bag and threw them on the open fire at home when no one was looking.

It is only now, more than forty years later, that I have talked to old school friends about this and discovered they were doing exactly the same.

Periods were briefly described in sex education lessons when we were thirteen, which must have been too late for many of the girls, but they were obviously still news to some of the boys. One of them turned around, appalled, on hearing about this monthly bleed, to look me and my three friends up and down as we sat on the row behind, shuddered and said, 'Urggh!'

Thirty years later, during my daughter's high school sex education lesson, things were not much different. On hearing the phrase 'vaginal fluids', one ashen-faced boy put up his hand to say he felt dizzy, and the teacher made him spend the rest of the class flat on the floor with his feet higher than his head.

Fortunately, my daughters were better prepared than I had been because I stumbled upon a copy of Claire Rayner's *The Body Book* in a charity shop and gave it to them while they were still at primary school. The cover showed two naked cartoon children standing in a cartoon pastoral idyll and gave clear details about puberty, conception, childbirth, life and death. My mother was wryly amused to see one of my daughters, then aged seven, write her letter to Father Christmas asking for a 'Professor Snape Potions Lab' then, after posting the letter up the chimney, go back to reading about vaginas and penises.

But at thirteen my body was a mystery to me. Despite the embarrassed science teacher drawing wombs and ovaries and Fallopian tubes on the blackboard in first-year science lessons, I could not grasp how the inside and the outside matched up. Until I gave birth myself, I didn't know a uterus was another name for a womb, nor the difference between a vulva and a vagina.

When I decided to try tampons rather than pads aged fifteen, those sex education lessons were no help. I daren't try Tampax because they looked unfeasibly huge – I didn't realise part of it was an applicator that didn't have to be inserted.

First, I had to 'borrow' some tampons from my elder sister, because I was too embarrassed to buy any. Why did corner shops keep them behind a counter, so you had to actually ask for them by name? I couldn't voice the word 'tampon' *out loud*. Plus, they were expensive (and taxed, although I didn't realise that at the time).

At least 'period poverty' – the problem of women and girls being too poor to access sanitary products – has improved for my daughters' generation, since the Scottish Government became the first in the world to make period products available free, including in schools.

Anyway, on first purloining a box of Lil-lets, I unfolded the tampon instructions and gazed at the drawn cross-section of the female body with its complicated tubes and openings and was terrified of inserting it in the wrong place. RELAX, said the instructions. It is IMPORTANT to RELAX. But what if the tampon went in too far? What if the string broke? What if I could not get it back out? What if it disappeared inside me completely?

If any of these catastrophes had happened, I would have been on my own because I would not have dared to tell anyone. It was around this time that I also first saw articles about toxic shock syndrome – a potentially fatal condition caused by tampons.

RELAX yelled the tampon instructions.

Information on women's bodies had been scarce ever since I got Diane, my first Tiny Tears doll, to discover it had only one hole, for peeing, at the back. If you fed her water from a bottle, it dripped from this rear hole. Presumably, the solitary peeing hole between the doll's bum cheeks had been some designer's decision – to keep real female anatomy well and truly out of it.

Ten

A 'Save the Date' for a wedding in Italy, in Cello's ancestral village, had been hanging on our kitchen dresser for a year, but the lumpectomy operation was scheduled for the same week.

If I did not go, Cello wouldn't go, and Lara would have to go alone. How miserable to be on a cancer ward rather than at a sunny Italian wedding.

A friend advised me to cancel the trip and get treated as soon as possible – but having cancer had made opportunities like this more precious.

I postponed the operation for a week, committed to going to the wedding, and hoped I didn't come to regret it.

Before the diagnosis I had bought two new bikinis – the first in thirty years – and had had a dress altered that had belonged to my little sister, Tricia. After Tricia died, we discovered a room full of beautiful clothes we didn't know she had. One of the dresses was black satin with gold and red orchids. I tried to slim into it but even a stone down it was too tight. I took it to a dressmaker in Edinburgh who could work miracles and she fitted invisible black satin inserts under the arms. I tried it on in the shop and she stood there, pins stuck between her clenched teeth, murmuring, 'Perfetto, perfetto'.

I packed the dress along with the Ruby Woo lipstick, but wondered if I would be able to ignore the cancer for five days or whether I would wish I had stayed at home to get the operation over with.

As soon as we arrived in Italy, I knew I had done the right thing. Scores of guests turned up by plane, train and bus at this beautiful place on the Golfo di Policastro for three days' relaxation before the wedding. The sea was blue, the sky was bluer and the sun was blazing. The food was divine. On a first night in Italy I like to sit by the sea, drink local wine and eat a bowl of olives – and never have they tasted so good. A giddy sense of celebration and of being away from home was drowning out the worry. I realised, exhilarated, that I had jumped off Planet Cancer for five days.

On the first evening, a troupe of entertainers streamed into the bar wearing embroidered traditional costume, yelling *Arriva! Arriva!*

'What are they saying?' I asked Cello. 'He's coming, he's coming,' he replied, and the hysteria that had been brewing since we arrived bubbled over and Lara and I laughed until we cried.

The troupe banged tambourines off their heads, leaping, dancing, smiling, singing, clapping, as all the Italians joined in with feeling, one dancing past with a plastic beach chair. The Brits watched with rictus grins, lost for words at this larger-than-life joyfulness, until eventually the troupe departed, still singing as they wended their way out of the restaurant, and then the more inhibited among us began to relax and tap our feet to the remaining backing track. 'I didn't think I was going to make it,' said Lara, 'I thought that was how I was going to die', and I laughed so hard I couldn't eat my rice ball.

One evening, the mother of the bride beckoned me over to her table to meet another guest. 'This is Christine,' she said, 'she has been through it too.' Christine was an elegant woman with a blonde bob. She smiled and pulled her top askew and pointed to a blue mark on her chest. 'From the radiotherapy,' she said.

I found it difficult to know how to react. I was not used to cancer being a part of me; it took me aback that people looked at me and thought 'cancer'. I was reluctant to be dragged away from the festivities and back to Planet Cancer, but Christine was a gracious, open, friendly woman, who was happy to share her experience. She showed me a photograph of herself on her phone, exhausted and bald from chemotherapy, very different from the glamorous woman in front of me.

Once again, I felt gratitude for the women who had hacked a path through the breast cancer jungle, ahead of me, and were willing to show me the way.

Next morning, I donned one of the new bikinis, only to overdo it on the first day, and end up at the wedding in the satin orchid dress with a fiery chest to match the Ruby Woo lipstick. It didn't matter. Excitement was high. The sea of tartan kilts in red, purple and green, at this Scots-Italian wedding, was causing a stir. As we left the hotel, a cycle race was delayed as skinny men in Lycra clamoured to take photographs.

We wound our way, in a convoy of buses, up the dizzying hair-pin bends that stretched the seven kilometres from the sea up to the village of Santa Marina – the family home of the father of the bride. We alighted in the lower piazza with views back down the forested mountainside to the sea.

I felt wonderful. Mainly because I was there at all, but also because I had been privy to the secret of Room 68. My hair had been put into an up-do that morning by a lady who spoke no English but who had arrived at the hotel armed with a comb, a bag of hair pins, industrial-strength hairspray and a ferocious grip. The whisper went round: 'She's in Room 68.' All it took was a picture of a hairdo from Instagram for the lady to study, nod and it was yours. My fascinator was fixed so firmly I thought it might never come off.

It was early September and the sun was strong on the white-washed houses as we left the buses behind and completed the climb up the tiny cobbled streets to the chapel. One hundred and fifty brightly coloured, glittering, chattering wedding guests. We passed the village water pump where the street got narrower and the houses got smaller – some with doorways so tiny the inhabitants must have to bend to get inside. Local people peered round doors and through dangling plastic fly-strips to watch this invasion. One woman dashed to bring in her washing, ripping down pillowcases and underwear, before the wedding party passed her front yard.

We were overtaken by Chris, the groom, and two groomsmen zooming by, kilts swaying, standing in the back of one of the three-wheeler trucks that navigate the tiny roads in mountainous Italian villages. This one was festooned with pink ribbons and tulle bows and balloons marked *Tanti Auguri!* ('Best Wishes!'). Horns blared, there were shouts and cheers, and over the whole experience there hung a feeling of unreality. I was living in a film set.

Maybe *this* was what I had meant by 'jumping off the world'.

The Chiesa Madre, the 'mother church', was packed, with guests spilling into the tiny ivy-clad piazza outside, where white-haired old ladies, dressed head to foot in black, watched from between tumbling red geraniums on iron balconies high overhead. The inside of the chapel belied the simplicity of the outside; the interior walls were sunshine yellow decorated with ornate white mouldings and archways, icons and paintings. Overhead were golden ceiling roses. The pews were full of fluttering white fans, like the wings of gigantic cabbage whites, as guests tried to cool themselves. From my position at the back, the hatinators and fascinators looked like a flock of exotic birds. The bridesmaids and bride's mother arrived sparkling and rosy pink and the happiness swelled.

Time stood still as we waited for the bride; the heat, the setting, the heightened emotion all adding to the surreal atmosphere in this place where generations of Cello's family stories have been absorbed into the stone.

Then the heart-lifting sound of pipers playing 'Highland

Cathedral' as the bride, Carla, arrived in a dress so exuberant, so joyous, with frills upon frills, that she and her father, Giovanni, could fit through the door and down the aisle thanks only to Giovanni's nifty sidestep. People turned, several jumped into the aisle for a photo, others craned for a better look, and then a great cheer erupted, lasting the entire walk to the altar.

I felt a grip on my throat. I could hardly breathe. My eyes stung. On the seat were individual packs of tissues labelled 'For Your Happy Tears'. I wasn't sure that my tears were entirely happy, but I was so glad to be there and to be sharing this moment – it was as though the whole spectacle was building to a crescendo to give me the bravery to carry me forward for what was to come.

On the last evening of the holiday, one of the guests twirled her champagne glass and remarked to Lara that she had hoped to lose so much weight for the wedding that people would think she was ill. Lara gazed at her speechless, before coming over to tell me: 'You'll never guess...'

Cello met someone he had not seen for years. I saw them having an intense conversation and I wandered across the restaurant to join them. The man was telling Cello about his wife, who had been diagnosed with breast cancer, but it had not been treated quickly enough and the disease had now spread to her brain. Cello translated the story for me from Italian. The social smile dropped from my face. The man looked at me, pointing at his head, tapping it urgently, *Fa lo presto, Fa lo presto,* he said, 'Get it done. Get it done quick.' It was like a terrifying crash-landing back to reality. It was time to go home and deal with it.

The day after returning from Italy, I went to the Western General Hospital Breast Clinic for my pre-op checks. I have always dreaded the Western General (known as 'The Western') because of its association with cancer. I did not think of it as a place of cures and healing but of suffering and death, despite its good reputation.

I had been sent a map of the hospital and my eyes scanned it. There was the Breast Clinic, and around it those dreaded words: Oncology, Palliative Care, Chaplaincy, Cancer Centre, Chemotherapy, Radiotherapy, Bereavement Suite, there was even a memorial garden. To be fair to the Western, there were also canteens and clock towers, libraries, shops and discharge lounges – but at that moment I couldn't register those.

When I arrived, there was another giant map of the hospital on the roadside. **You Are Here**, it said, and an arrow pointed to the Department of Clinical Oncology and the Breast Unit, all coloured-in mucky-brown. **You Are Here**.

I know I am here, I thought. It was still hard to believe I was here. I almost expected to find an addendum: **You Are Here. You didn't expect this, did you?**

The nurse in the Breast Clinic weighed and measured me as though I was off to meet the hangman. Cello asked who would do the operation. Were they experienced? She tapped on her keyboard and gave us his name. He was very experienced, she assured us. I wondered if they ever informed anyone that no, as a matter of fact, he's fresh out of surgeon school – never done this sort of thing before in his life.

She chuckled to herself about the surgeon; told us he was a tease. I was not sure what to do with that information.

'He may inject your breast with blue dye to help locate the lymph nodes,' she warned. 'Don't be alarmed if you wake up with a blue face or pass blue water.'

She also told me to bring a dressing gown and slippers, and a non-underwired bra – and it was these last trivial details that threw me.

Ten

I did not own a dressing gown or slippers, or a non-underwired bra, and I resented deeply having to buy a dressing gown and slippers and a non-underwired bra for *cancer*.

With only a day to get ready, I trudged off into the city centre to browse non-underwired bras – frumpy items I associated with young girls and old ladies, although at my size, 34F, the bras I was looking at were more likely to be for old ladies who had abandoned all idea of uplift. I chose two, hanging vastly on plastic hangers, looking like something from the Second World War, possibly called 'utility brassieres', or maybe items designed by a Soviet committee.

Resentment at this enforced shopping spree mounted.

I searched for a dressing gown and slippers that were not too expensive or too heavy because hospitals are always hot. I found a silk dressing gown covered in pink and blue orchids in John Lewis. It was beautiful. It was also fifty pounds and I refused to pay fifty pounds for a *cancer* dressing gown.

At the Italian wedding, the bridal party had worn matching silk dressing gowns to get ready – but that was for a wedding, not for *cancer*.

In Primark there was a see-through thing with a cartoon dog. No point in a see-through thing. Didn't want a cartoon dog. In TK Maxx, they were big and fluffy – too big, too fluffy. I turned to the assistant who was hanging up complicated sleepwear, all lace and thin straps tangled in a cat's cradle.

'I need a lightweight dressing gown for hospital. I've got cancer.'

'Oh dear,' she said, still gripping a lace strap between her teeth. She nodded towards the big and fluffy items. ''Fraid that's all we've got.'

I phoned Cello, frustrated, upset, furious. How difficult could it be to buy a dressing gown?

'Get the fifty-pound one,' he said. 'Do you want me to buy it for you?'

No! *No I did not*! I have never been good at spending money on myself and I was *not* going to start with a fifty-pound *cancer* dressing gown.

I marched around the shop blinded by tears. Why hadn't I realised I would need a dressing gown? Why was I so stupid? Storming down the street I was engulfed by utter fury: I did not want cancer; I did not want to spend time and energy and money on cancer. I did not want to have any dealings with cancer *at all*. I wanted the whole horrible cancer thing to go away and leave me alone.

I phoned my brother-in-law, Marino, a travel guide who spends half his life in five-star hotels, and he offered me some new hotel slippers. 'Black, red or white?' he asked.

I accepted the free slippers, asking for the black – black was the only colour suitable for cancer slippers – but I vowed I would *never* buy a *cancer* dressing gown.

Instead, I walked the one hundred yards from TK Maxx to the Scottish National Portrait Gallery because art galleries soothe me even in the fraughtest of times.

The doors were flung open by a tartan-clad doorman with a big smile. Usually, I crossed the echoing mosaic floor and headed past the columns covered in gold leaf, past the white marble Rabbie Burns, through the lintel carved with 'The National Museum of Antiquities', up two flights of stairs, turning right past James Naughtie, Denise Mina and Rikki Fulton, and then I would sit on one of the leather cubes, under the eye of Norman MacCaig, to stare at my favourite painting, one I have visited regularly for years and which never fails to fascinate: *Three Oncologists* by Ken Currie.

This painting is ethereal and haunted. It shows Prof. R. J.

Steele, Prof. Sir Alfred Cuschieri and Prof. Sir David Lane, of the Department of Surgery and Molecular Oncology at Ninewells Hospital in Dundee. These men appear to have been disturbed in the middle of carrying out cancer operations and have blood on their hands. They glance over their shoulders, out of the frame, looking weighed down, exhausted, apprehensive and wary. They appear to be not quite of this world, hovering somewhere between life and death. They are luminous against a dark curtained background as though they are forming a barrier between this world and the next, but are unsure whether, or for how long, they can keep up the fight.

Usually, I would sit and look at this painting, from face to haunted face.

But today I hesitated beside the tartan-clad doorman and instead of heading upstairs, I took a sharp right into the café. I bought a scone and coffee and sat under the steely eye of Muriel Spark to think about the *Three Oncologists*. In a notice pinned beside the painting upstairs, Ken Currie says: 'I want the viewer to be simultaneously attracted and repulsed by my work in the same glance. My aim is to provoke anxiety and discomfort in the act of looking – to hold their gaze then mercilessly unsettle them.'

I knew I could not face the *Three Oncologists* today; I was anxious, discomforted and mercilessly unsettled enough.

I finished my scone, gulped my coffee, and headed home to pack.

The Admission Instructions was the usual joyless list: *Please do not eat or chew gum after midnight on the evening prior to admission … you may drink up to 2 small cups of still water, but no fizzy or flavoured water, prior to 6am … ALL patients are required to bring dressing gown and slippers…*

I shoved a bobbly full-length grey cardie into the bag in place of a dressing gown.

I am not sure who or what I was trying to defy.

Cello sent me an email headed: 'No complaints about surgeon.' He had Googled 'name of my surgeon + complaint'. Just in case.

I spoke to my friend, Mandy, who herself had been under observation at the Western Breast Unit. When I told her who my surgeon was, she was excited: 'Oooh, he's mine too, I love him! He's gorgeous and so charming.' She laughed. 'I put my best black bra on when I have an appointment with him. My husband gets jealous.'

To kill time, I decided to write a poem. I opened my notebook and jotted down 'Googling My Oncologist'. I slowly underlined the words 'Googling My Oncologist' and considered how the two words you never want to meet are 'My' and 'Oncologist'.

That evening, I was supposed to read from my unpublished memoir in public, for the first time. I had been invited to give a talk to my home village in Lancashire, where the book is based – which seemed an appropriate place for it to be born. I was to give a talk in the village hall following their annual harvest festival supper of hotpot and apple pie. But it was a four-hour journey and this after-dinner speaking date, which had been in the diary for months, had fallen on the night between the pre-op checks and the operation. I was stressed about this; I hated letting people down and I resented cancer making me unreliable.

My nephew, Christopher, an inspector in the Metropolitan Police, had taken leave to come and hear me speak. When I told him I wasn't going to be able to make it, he replied, 'What's your Plan B?' To which I replied, 'You are.' So, that evening, as I packed my bag in Edinburgh, the people of my home village were listening to a talk about modern policing in London, and the debut for my memoir would have to wait.

Instead, I stood in front of the bedroom mirror naked from

the waist up. Should I take a 'before' picture? The skin on my chest was a golden brown from the Italian sun. The skin that had been hidden under the new bikini a startling white by comparison. There was a faint scar from the biopsy seven weeks ago. What would I look like after this operation? Would I be symmetrical? Would I be lopsided? Would I be numb? Would I be badly scarred? How many scars would there be?

I decided not to take a picture, so it didn't flash up next time I printed my photos off in Boots.

I took a last look at myself.

There was still no outward sign of the cancer, no lump and no pain, which made it difficult to grasp that the cells in my right breast had turned against me.

I was entering another era in the history of my body.

Eleven

I have had breasts for forty-five years and it has been complicated.

I remember running across one of our fields with a boy cousin when I was seven years old. From a distance, fields appear to be flat and made for running, but they are not – they have divots made by cows' hooves, they have deep puddles, cow pats, thistles, nettles and unexpected rises and falls, but as a child I was fast and lean, and I could fly across this field; nothing could stop me. I knew I could keep up with my cousin, even though he was older than me. In my mind, to 'run like a girl' was a good thing.

I glanced sideways, watching him racing along beside me, and I was so glad I had nothing flopping between my legs – how annoying to be a boy, I thought. How could they enjoy running? How wonderful to be a girl and feel the freedom of nothing jiggling when you moved.

I loved to stand on my hands against the privet hedge, to dangle upside-down on a rope, to do somersaults on the hay bales, and leap from the swing in the garden when it was so high the chains had gone slack. I was in control of my body; it was lean and taut. I enjoyed that it did what I wanted.

What a shock I was in for.

This was the 1970s and a lot of television light entertainment was sexualised in a nudge-nudge wink-wink kind of way. Women's bodies were funny, it seemed. Breasts were comic props, as were long legs in short skirts, especially up a ladder. We laughed as Benny Hill chased big-busted women in hot pants – his 'Angels' apparently – round and round to a silly tune, leering knowingly as he passed the camera, signalling to other men 'we're all in on *this* joke'.

We laughed when Barbara Windsor's bra flew off in *Carry on Camping*. We watched *Casanova 73*, 'The adventures of a 20th-century libertine', written by Galton & Simpson, in which a sleazy Leslie Phillips, a 'successful businessman and compulsive philanderer', also leered for laughs at women's breasts and up women's skirts.

We laughed at Miss Brahms in *Are You Being Served?*, whose breasts and legs were often the butt of the joke. She was played by Wendy Richards who, in 1986, almost overnight, morphed from the sex object Miss Brahms into hard-faced matriarch Pauline Fowler in *EastEnders*. Miss Brahms was sidekick to hyper-sexualised Mrs Slocombe, thirty years her senior, who was depicted as sexually frustrated, cat-loving and unable to speak without uttering a double-entendre: 'I've got a sculptor coming this evening, he's going to do my pussy in clay.'

We watched every secretary in every sitcom being portrayed as a something called a 'dolly bird', bending over the boss's desk and being ogled and leched over. These women were nothing like my dollies, which were armless, legless, with shorn hair and drawn-on glasses; no, these dolly birds were pert, giggly, bouffant, slim and a bit daft.

The phrase 'dolly birds' – young women who were sexy but stupid – sums up seventies' light entertainment. In the world of television – which to us was the real world – breasts and brains did not mix. These female characters, dead behind the eyes and with no more personality than blow-up dolls, were not fully human.

Sometimes the dolly birds were also 'beautiful assistants', so while middle-aged Bruce Forsyth capered and gurned on *The Generation Game*, his twenty-one-year-old 'beautiful assistant' (and later, wife) Anthea Redfern didn't do much more than glide on stage while wearing a frock: *Give us a twirl, Anthea!* Likewise, Bob Monkhouse regularly wise-cracked on *The Golden Shot* that *his* beautiful assistant, twenty-one-year-old Anne Aston, could not add up. *Anne Aston can't count to two unless she lifts up her jumper!* Another example of pretty + buxom = stupid.

In our household, like in many homes, the television was never turned off in the evenings. As a ten-year-old, I watched it and took it all in, but did not have the knowledge or the words to understand what was really being said. The seventies were an 'Ooh er matron' era and a strange time to grow up. Maybe it is always a strange time to grow up for girls.

We took Miss World seriously, thinking Miss Venezuela or Miss Mexico, having paraded with rictus grins in their 'swim-wear', had been officially declared the most beautiful woman in the world – somebody called Eric Morley in a bow tie said so. Miss World symbolised what I wanted to be: beautiful, admired and wearing a crown.

Twenty-five million viewers watched agog as the beauty queens' 'vital statistics' were read out: Miss Guam, 35 23 35, Miss Honduras 37 24 38. These statistics clearly were 'vital' – being the most important details about them.

A year or two later I joined the Bay City Rollers Fan Club and in my 'Membership Pack', besides a letter from Manager Tam Paton (*Always Yours, Tam X*), I received an information sheet giving me the 'measurements' of each Roller – 'Eric: Chest 36", Waist 28", Collar Size 14", Eyes blue' – but those were 'measure-ments' and did not seem 'vital'. Anyway, I was more interested in Eric's preferences for 'Peach Flambé, Ferraris and Benny Hill'.

In 1970, when Women's Lib protesters invaded the Miss World stage, throwing flour bombs and leaflets at Bob Hope in his tux, yelling, 'We are liberationists! We're not beautiful, we're not ugly, we're angry', with signs reading *If you want meat go to the butchers*, my sisters and I thought, 'Stop spoiling the fun, we want to see the long frocks.'

I noted the sneer in the way the television presenter said the phrase 'Women's Lib', but had no understanding of what it meant.

To be a beauty queen in the sexualised yet moralistic seventies, your reputation had to be 'unsullied'. In 1974, Miss UK had to resign her Miss World title after four days because it was revealed she was an 'unmarried mother'. I felt her gut-wrenching disappointment at having to hand back that crown of wire and paste.

When I heard my older cousins calling breasts 'bommers' I didn't make the connection between the things under ladies' blouses and war planes, until I eventually realised: 'Oh, *bombers*!' We pulled our jumpers out in two cones, put on our mother's high heels, and said, 'Look at *my* bombers.' At primary school, we laughed as one girl's bombers bounced when she danced around the maypole. After all, bombers were funny, right?

Meanwhile, my Tressy doll (a less popular Barbie) was the picture of elegance with her perpetual high-heeled feet, her wasp waist and her perky bombers with the nipple holes we made with a needle. She was an 'inaction' figure; only good for marrying Cousin John's Action Man when Cousin John was not there. Action Man had gripping hands for his grenades, back packs, guns and helmets, and could dangle from his cross-living-room zip wire, but furious Cousin John made him divorce Tressy every single time he found out, despite Tressy's shapely figure in her white wedding dress. *Action Man DOES NOT get married!*

The only kind of breasts in real life were our mothers' and grandmothers' 'busts', which were like bolsters, covered in cardigans and pinnies and the same all the way across.

It was different when bombers grew for real. Then they became boobs to girls, and tits, jugs, bazookas, baps, knockers, bristols or melons to boys – undignified, comic names thrown about to exert the power of embarrassment over the girls.

In my experience, breasts grew quickly and without warning, leaving you self-conscious and with no time to acclimatise to your new environment. My body was no longer taut, it was becoming decidedly untaut, with soft bits and bulging bits that at first, as a ten-year-old, I fully expected to disappear again.

Breasts apparently sent out signals about who you were, but the signals were in a code you hadn't mastered and were impossible to turn off. You got a 'trainer bra'. Training for what? Were the breasts being trained, or were you?

Breasts were to be covered and disguised. The baggier the clothes the better – even if big jumpers made you look like a sack of potatoes.

At high school I wore a home-made grey cardigan buttoned up with enormous toggles throughout the scorching summer of 1976, until a history teacher interrupted his lesson on 'Ship Design in Nelson's Navy' to leer, 'How hot has it got to get before you take off that cardigan?' The class laughed. It got to over ninety degrees Fahrenheit, but I never took it off.

I was left feeling I had made an immoral choice by acquiring breasts. *Tut, tut, but you* did *choose a showy pair. How vulgar.*

There was shame attached to them – some sort of moral judgement. As my breasts grew, I let my fringe grow over my face so I could hide behind it and I became round-shouldered to shrink and hide, unwittingly taking up the classic stance of the shamed, with downcast eyes and slack posture.

'We all know why the boys like *you*,' said a girl at school, despite the disguise of my ever-present grey cardie.

I wasn't even aware the boys *did* like me – although I knew I got unwanted attention from some who liked to point and discuss loudly whether they could see the shape of a girl's nipples through her cotton school shirt – *nipples! nipples!* – which was another reason for the grey cardie.

School swimming lessons were also mortifying – all that getting changed behind too-small towels, struggling in and out of clothing in a tiny communal changing room trying not to expose any body parts, then afterwards, writhing, still damp and reeking of chlorine, back into your uniform.

PE was just as bad, clamping your elbows across your chest to stop the wobbling and the bouncing as you were forced through the motions of some pointless team game. Then the horror of the communal shower, which must have been an exercise in humiliation and power by the teachers because it certainly wasn't an exercise in getting clean. The teacher's only concern being that you went in the shower naked, not whether you washed. Drop your towels! *Drop! Your! Towels!*

'Them teachers are just big old lezzers,' declared my fourteen-year-old cousin.

A classmate, who was called 'Fatso' by the PE teacher while doing Keep Fit to 'Forever in Blue Jeans' by Neil Diamond, became too self-conscious to use the communal showers and was taken into the teacher's office: 'Everyone else is going in the showers, what's so *different* about *you?*'

It says a lot about the trauma of the occasion that forty-five years later she still remembers the exact song that was playing.

I found everything about school sports loathsome. It taught me I couldn't do things. It taught me that sport was not for me.

A few years after leaving school, a boyfriend and I took a duvet to the middle of the school running track and had sex there at midnight as a final 'fuck you' to the PE department.

Breasts made appearances in books in my early teens, too, including *Carrie* by Stephen King, a book about the terrors of living in a young girl's body with its ability to change and become monstrous. As Carrie gets ready for prom, her mother looks at her dress and gasps, 'I can see your dirty pillows. Everyone will.' And Carrie replies, 'Those are my breasts, Momma. Every woman has them.'

Indeed they did, but some breasts were more troublesome than others.

Big breasts (and tiny waists) featured in 1970s bodice rippers – books as thick as bricks with names like *Sweet Savage Love*, a title that was passed around half the girls in my class in 1976 and even some of their mothers; books with front covers showing women with ripped dresses and half their breasts exposed as they were tied to a stake or lashed to a horse by a man in a mask. Books I thought were about adventure and romance but, thirty-five years later, I realise were about kidnap and rape. The heaving, tousled heroine of *Sweet Savage Love* was described as 'beautiful, impudent and innocent'. No wonder we were confused.

On the school bus I saw a girl get her arms fastened behind her back by two boys as another boy groped her breasts. All of the bullies on the back seat laughed. The girl laughed too as though she was in on the joke, but we all knew better.

Several times I heard the 'joke' 'More than a handful's a waste', which implied breasts were for the pleasure of others and I had made an unwise choice by acquiring breasts that were too big.

Breasts were here and they brought a lot of baggage and pitfalls with them.

It seemed a long, long time since I could run so fast and free that I felt I could fly.

One Saturday evening when I was thirteen the nation chortled with glee as Penelope Keith – the posh actress from the sitcom *The Good Life* – said the word 'fart' on the *Parkinson* show. I remember the audience exploding with laughter. Maybe I recall it so clearly because I was being molested at the time. A family friend, someone I thought of as a big brother, was groping my breasts, through my home-made cotton nightie – a baggy garment with a gathered neck like something out of *Little House on the Prairie*. Then he unzipped his jeans, took his penis out and squeezed my hand round it as I froze, saying nothing. Meanwhile, my parents slept unaware upstairs, Parky chuckled and the studio audience roared at a posh woman saying 'fart', because, apparently, *that* was taboo and shocking.

I was too ashamed to tell anyone. Maybe it was my fault for having breasts in the first place? And such obvious ones. After all, *Casanova 73* had warned what the upshot of having breasts was likely to be.

Forty-odd years later, I searched for that clip of Michael Parkinson interviewing Penelope Keith. Only part of the interview was available online and I couldn't find the fart joke – just endless minutes of Parkinson asking Penelope Keith, 'You are tall, aren't you? Is it a problem being so tall? As a teen were you self-conscious about your height? Did it affect your relationship with the fellas? What do you do about small leading fellas? Aren't you tall!'

Getting too tall was a fear of mine; as a young teen I lay in the bath forcing the soles of my feet against the tap end and the top of my head against the round end, hoping my body would get the message to stop growing. I dreaded growing too big, taking up too much space, becoming 'manly'. Although whether that was before or after the Parkinson interview, I can't remember. At thirteen, all I wanted to do was fit in, to conform, to do what I was 'supposed' to do, to be the same as everyone else, not to draw attention to myself – but having big breasts made that impossible.

A baggy cotton nightie had obviously not been enough protection.

Two years later, when I went to my first concert – The Boomtown Rats at Lancaster University – I squeezed onto the parcel shelf of my sister's friend's MG wearing a chunky-knit polo neck. 'You'll get too hot,' the friend said. 'Haven't you got a T-shirt?' No, I said, I did not have a T-shirt. I did not own a T-shirt. Wearing a T-shirt when you had grown-up breasts was as exposing as going out in your underwear.

I sweltered through the concert, hanging out at the back protected by mounds of wool, watching other girls screaming and fainting as Bob Geldof sang 'Mary of the 4th Form' – a song about an over-sexualised schoolgirl who 'turns all the boys on' by doing the apparently controversial: sitting at her desk, opening her mouth and picking up her pencil. The song implies that schoolgirl Mary abuses her sexual power over 'natural' adult men – but from where I was standing, in my knitted armour, being in the fourth form did not feel powerful at all. I was shy, naïve, introverted, keen to please and in a constant state of discomfort and embarrassment caused by acute self-consciousness. This was not an empowering combination for a fifteen-year-old.

The following year, Joe Jackson sang 'It's Different for Girls', and I wondered if he knew *how* different.

Having two daughters showed me that things had not changed much in the policing of young women and their bodies by the time they got to secondary school in the 2000s. A male teacher told my fourteen-year-old daughter's class, 'It's not about whether girls are showing too much, it's about whether I am uncomfortable.' Another female teacher – a self-proclaimed feminist – told the girls, 'Leave more to the imagination.' She ordered Lara to the front of the class and told her to pick up a pencil in her short skirt, to see if she could do so decently. Lara refused.

But although girls can choose whether they expose skin or not - and what they 'leave to the imagination' in that sense – they cannot choose whether they have breasts or not. They cannot choose their physical shape.

As it had for me thirty years before, the very fact of having breasts bigger than her peers made my daughter, Lara, feel 'unacceptable'. Her flat-chested friends could wear vest tops and leggings in the park without comment, whereas when she wore them the boys shouted, 'Getting your boobs out again?' or sang the Katy Perry lyrics, 'Tight jeans, double Ds'. Her natural shape made her a vulnerable, blame-worthy target. In a re-run of my grey cardie disguise from 1976, my daughter bought shirts several sizes too big for protection.

Shaming girls for their appearance is an everyday occurrence in schools. When Lara was seventeen, she was standing in the corridor of her non-denominational school wearing lip gloss as the headteacher marched past and declared, 'You look like a painted Jezebel, and if you read the Bible you'd know that was an insult.' Lara did not read the Bible, so she consulted Google, then told her friend, 'I think the Head just called me a whore.'

On another occasion, he yelled at her across a crowded corridor, 'You're wearing false eyelashes – that's against school uniform. Go home and remove them.' Lara stopped a passing female teacher to verify that her eyelashes were in fact natural.

'She's Italian. They're hers!'

Lara believes this nit-picking about eyelashes and lip gloss was an excuse to pick on and shame girls. 'You were between a rock and a hard place, either bullied by other pupils for not wearing make-up or bullied by the teachers for wearing it.'

I tried to teach my daughters to speak up for themselves more effectively than I had as a tongue-tied teenager. As a result, Nina was voted 'Rudest Member of the Class' and Lara was in her yearbook as 'The One with the Biggest Ego' – speaking up by girls is not always welcomed.

Throughout my high school years, 1975–1980, the North-West of England was terrorised by Peter Sutcliffe, the serial killer who became known as the Yorkshire Ripper.

His presence loomed larger as the years passed and more details became known of how he sneaked up behind women and hit them over the head with hammers, stabbed them, sexually assaulted them, and desecrated their bodies.

In 1979, my school friends and I listened to the tape of the killer taunting the police. *You are no nearer catching me now than you were five years ago when I started.* The tape was made available to the public via a 'Dial-the-Ripper' hotline in an attempt to identify him. In fact, the tape was a hoax, but it felt very real to us as we listened to it in a public phone box and screamed in terror at hearing what we believed to be his voice – throwing the telephone receiver to each other like a hot potato. *I don't want it! I don't want it!*

In September 1980, the police warned women in the North-West not to go out alone at night because they believed he was due to murder again. My friend, Hilary, and I went on an A-Level English trip from Preston (where a woman's murder had mistakenly been put down to Sutcliffe) to Manchester (where he had already murdered two). We headed off on a coach to the Royal Exchange Theatre to see Helen Mirren in the violent revenge tragedy *The Duchess of Malfi*.

After watching Helen Mirren say, 'Pull and pull strongly' as her murderers approached with ropes to strangle her, for not doing what she was told, we headed home. Hilary's portable tape deck played 'Howzat, you messed around, I caught you out, howzat' as we peered out, at the back yards and byways of town after town, wondering if he was out there, wondering which back alley he was prowling down now, but seeing little more than our own anxious expressions reflected back to us in the coach window.

During the following days and weeks, Sutcliffe attacked three more women, who survived, then two months later he murdered Jacqueline Hill, a twenty-year-old English student in Leeds. He was eventually convicted of murdering thirteen women and attacking ten more.

It seemed that danger to women was everywhere, woven into the fabric of art and life.

Twelve

Early on the day of the operation, Cello drove me to the Oncology Department and stayed with me until I was moved to a 'Female Only' area and he could go no further.

I waved him goodbye, clinging to my phone like a lifeline.

There were six beds in the ward and on each bed, placed under the *Nil by Mouth* signs, were handmade, heart-shaped cushions. On my bed, the cushion was yellow and blue, with a note attached from a local sewing group: *Made with care and attention just for you...* A nurse demonstrated how the cushion would fit under my arm to protect my wound.

I perched on the chair beside my bed – a 'day bed' – which appeared to mean a very narrow bed indeed. Nurses bustled about and several times they asked, 'Have you been admitted? Have you signed the consent forms?' To which the answer was always 'no'. Apparently, my surgeon would arrive at any minute to admit me and get me to sign the necessary paperwork.

I chatted to the lady in the next bed. Familiar questions: which breast? How big is your tumour? Is there breast cancer in your family? Was it a mammogram or did you find a lump? By now these stories were well-rehearsed.

A nurse rushed past: had my surgeon admitted me yet? Had I signed the forms? The answer was still no.

The ward was a strange mix of medical and homely. Efforts had been made to make it more welcoming than a normal ward and there was a juxtaposition of the medical with the personal. Real-life furniture with something of TK Maxx about it – a unit with bamboo drawers and paintings of flowers – were placed beside signs reading: *Management of needlestick and contamination Injuries.*

The nurse returned: had the surgeon admitted me and got me to sign the consent forms yet?

Unfortunately, the answer was still no.

The nurse attached claustrophobic wristbands as snug as handcuffs. I was given a hospital gown and some long white anti-embolism stockings, to stop blood clots forming – socks so tight I feared trapping my finger-ends as I wrangled them on. I pulled the curtain round my bed, removed my top and bra and wrapped myself in the back-fastening hospital gown. Not having a dressing gown, I put on my full-length grey cardie. The ward was freezing, and I remembered ruefully the rejected fluffy dressing gowns in TK Maxx. I tugged the cardie sleeves over my cold hands and got out my brother-in-law's freebie slippers, shoving my white-stockinged feet into the black plush slip-ons incongruously embossed in gold: 'Baglioni Hotels Five Star'.

I did not take off my jogging bottoms or pants. I felt vulnerable enough without removing any more clothing.

A different nurse appeared. Had my surgeon admitted me and got me to sign the consent forms yet?

Nope.

A young man arrived with a tea trolley; apparently my operation would not be until the afternoon, so I was allowed a cup of black tea. I gripped it with both hands, trying to stop myself shaking. Twenty minutes later a nurse joked, 'You're clinging on to that for dear life', and I realised that yes, I was.

There was discussion among the nurses; it was now pressing that I be admitted and sign the forms as I was due a preliminary procedure.

It seemed my surgeon was not around after all, so another surgeon came to admit me. He was friendly, Spanish, in his thirties. He perched on the bed and asked my name and date of birth and I signed the forms. He took a black sharpie and drew something across my right collar bone.

'What have you written?' I asked. 'This one, with a downward arrow?'

He smiled as though he didn't hear that every day.

No, he explained, he had written WLE, meaning 'wide local excision'. This was another name for a lumpectomy and meant the tumour would be removed along with some surrounding healthy tissue. I was also to have a 'sentinel node biopsy', which meant removing the first lymph node the cancer would drain into to see if the cancer had spread, plus several more lymph nodes.

I latched onto this man's friendliness, having been left nervous and vulnerable by my surgeon's no-show, which felt like a failure on my part. All of the other women had been admitted ages ago. We chatted a bit and I said how much I appreciated the touch with the cushions. He nodded and said, 'People ask me: why breast surgery?, and I tell them it's ... *nicer*.'

It was now 10.30am and I needed to get a wire inserted into the tumour because the cancer did not form a palpable lump and the surgeon would need guidance to find it in the operating theatre.

I had been warned about this possibility during the pre-op meeting, but it had sounded so brutal and primitive – a wire inserted? An *actual* wire? Into the cancer? I had hoped it would not happen; that there would be a higher-tech way. But no.

A nurse took me and the woman in the next bed downstairs to the mammography department. We sat in the corridor; she in her enviably warm and fluffy dressing gown, me in my long cardie, and we discussed what a shock it had been. One of us said, 'I couldn't believe it', and the other nodded, 'neither could I', and we both silently stared at the wall.

I was taken to get the wire inserted. Remembering how painful the needle biopsy had been, I decided that this time more information might help. I asked the doctor to show me the wire she would insert. Maybe to see it would demystify the process and reduce my anxiety. She held up a surprisingly long, thick, dark wire. It looked like something from my gardening basket, and I realised I had been expecting thin, silver five-amp fuse wire. 'This is the wire,' she said, adding, 'I will insert it into the breast by threading it into this hollow needle', and she held up a needle device so thick it made me feel sick. That was too big. How could that be described as a needle?

Maybe knowledge is not always power.

My breathing had become shallow with fear. I told her about the agonising biopsy, and she promised to inject me with plenty of anaesthetic.

After she had done so, she used an ultrasound to find the tumour, guide the needle and insert the wire. I gazed determinedly in the opposite direction, and she chatted casually with her colleague as if this was an everyday occurrence (which to her, of course, it was).

Afterwards, I glanced down at my breast and, despite knowing it would be there, I was alarmed to see wire sticking out of me, bunched up, maybe a foot long. I had expected the doctor to trim it short. Instead, she coiled it up neatly and stuck it down on my breast with a dressing.

Next was a mammogram to check the wire was in the right place. I removed my hospital gown to stand at the mammography machine naked from the waist up, but still wearing my jogging bottoms. The mammographer commented that sometimes women ended up coming for pre-op mammograms naked under their gowns. 'There's no need for it!' she said, and I agreed. It is impossible to be assertive with no knickers on.

It was a horrifying thought, having my breast crushed between two glass plates when there was a wire inserted in the flesh, but I forced myself not to look and was grateful the anaesthetic had not worn off.

I thought back to the mammogram that had kicked all this off three months before – how I had not been sure about having *one* mammogram and now here I was having lost count of all my mammograms.

Back in the ward, the woman in the next bed and I, with our matching dressings covering our wire inserts, discovered we had daughters of a similar age. Her daughter had recently married, mine had got engaged. She told me about wedding venues and hog roasts, ceilidhs and silent discos and for a few minutes life seemed almost normal. We eyed up the other patients' heart-shaped cushions: 'That red would go nice with my bedroom,' she muttered, nodding towards the woman in the corner with her poppy cushion, but I liked my blue and yellow one and patted it territorially.

One by one, the other women disappeared for surgery, until it was time for the woman in the next bed. I wished her luck and watched her being wheeled away. Then I was alone on the ward. Even the nurses had disappeared.

My 'Patient Information' suggested this would be a good time to 'relax until it is time to go to theatre', but I had never felt less relaxed in my life – this was worse than my first encounter with a tampon. I hadn't eaten for sixteen hours, but I was too frightened to be hungry.

I had brought books, but I could not read. People had kept recommending a best-selling memoir by a junior doctor. *It's hilarious! You'll love it!* But I had avoided that one, frightened it would be full of patients being mocked and ridiculed. I was too vulnerable for that. I had brought music, but I could not listen.

I sat on the low chair by my bed and felt as though I was slowly vanishing.

Then a man in a smart blue suit strode into the room. He was clearly an important man in a hurry. I recognised him as my consultant surgeon from the Google search. He glanced at me, said nothing and marched to the nurses' desk where he picked up a brown file of notes, which must have been mine – there were no other patients or notes in there. He flicked through and gave a loud sigh of irritation. Those notes were obviously not what he was looking for.

I urged myself to speak. Now was the opportunity to make a connection with the person about to operate on me. Say hello, introduce myself. It seemed important, but I could not utter a word.

He tossed the file back onto the desk and any opportunity to speak passed. He turned on his heel and marched from the room. I felt myself shrink even smaller; atom by atom I was sinking, disappearing into the low grey chair. The surgeon about to take a scalpel to me had not even acknowledged me and I was weighed down with dread.

My confidence was dragged even lower because I was sitting without make-up in a hospital gown. Who invented the hospital gown? Was it done to anonymise and render the patient as helpless as possible? I was grateful for my familiar grey cardie and I pulled it tight.

I was not exposed; it was not that my privacy was being denied, but the act of removing most of my own clothes and putting on this gown with 'Hospital Property' printed all over it in yellow, green and red had humbled me and put me at the bottom of the hierarchy. In this world – and it did feel like another world hermetically sealed – I had no role, no status, no badge, not even a trolley to push. My identity had been excised.

I was no longer me; I was a 'patient' – a word originally meaning 'one who suffers'. The hospital gown is a mark of that suffering, of stigma, like a hair shirt or a prison jumpsuit, the opposite of a business suit, the very opposite of power dressing. It is a tragicomic item; the only good place for a hospital gown is in a sitcom or a comedy sketch, and I was in neither. In my mind's ear I heard the signature tune to the seventies sitcom set on an NHS ward *Only When I Laugh* – a mournful rendition of 'I'm H.A.P.P.Y, I'm H.A.P.P.Y, I know I am, I'm sure I am, I'm H.A.P.P.Y'. I felt pathetic in the true sense of the word – someone to be pitied – and I did not like it.

A nurse strode in. 'Did he say hello?' she nodded in the direction of the vanished surgeon. I shook my head.

'What's he like?' she said, rolling her eyes, one hand on her hip, smiling fondly.

'Like a bastard,' I wanted to say, but I was mute.

To stop myself disappearing altogether and leaving nothing but a crumpled gown and anti-embolism socks, I grabbed my phone and messaged some friends.

'*My surgeon has walked in, bashed some folders about and marched out without saying a word (I know it's him cos Google). I'm hoping he's in a better mood when it's my turn.*'

I stared at the phone, watching the winking icon tell me: 'Someone is typing a reply', willing it to appear quicker. Being in contact with the outside world – having someone acknowledge me – was helping me regain a part of myself and fight the desire to flee the hospital.

I heard two nurses in the corridor, out of sight. They were making a bed and speculating about money donated to cancer charities: 'Where does it go?' asked one, 'that's what I wonder.' 'I know,' came the reply. 'What happened to that £90,000? I think if you want to help you need to give the money direct.' They continued in this vein for a few minutes until I heard shrieks of laughter: 'We've made the bed upside-down!'

I was dizzy with the desire to get out, to make a run for it, as far and as fast as I could – while at the same time fully aware there was a cancerous tumour in my breast speared on a wire and I was, in fact, all out of fleeing options.

Thirteen

Twenty-three years before my cancer operation, I had been marooned on the labour ward after giving birth for the first time. The maternity hospital was known as the 'Simpson Memorial', which was an odd name (for me, at least).

Then too I had the sensation of being reduced.

The labour suite – the room in which you give birth – was full of staff coming and going, talking and laughing at private jokes, yelling over my bed, continuing conversations begun in the corridor. It was a big room with activity happening all over the place in which I seemed to be incidental. The staff were described as a 'team', but it felt more like a gang of which I was not a member.

My waters had broken around midday on Saturday just as Cello settled down to watch *Football Focus*. I was admitted to hospital that afternoon, three weeks before my due date, armed optimistically with a bottle of Bach Rescue Remedy, Enya's *Watermark* on cassette tape and a birth plan, with a front cover showing a stork carrying a baby, in which I had written: 'I definitely want a painkilling epidural.' This was despite having attended antenatal classes where pain relief was looked down on and we were taught that a good birth was all in the breathing.

By 4am on Sunday – the Badlands if you want an anaesthetist – Enya was long gone, the Rescue Remedy forgotten, and I had been asking for an epidural since the day before. At first I was told, 'But you're doing so well…', then, hours later, despite many requests, I was informed, 'You've left it too late'.

I had been in labour for sixteen hours when one of the midwives – a loud, bossy woman who reminded me of my old PE teacher (it could have been the bright white trainers and the ponytail, or the barking orders and lack of compassion) – yelled across the room,

'You'd better get that baby out by half four or I'm going for the forceps', before catching her colleague's eye and smirking.

Clearly, she thought I wasn't trying hard enough, I wasn't cooperating, and the threat of a more violent birth would teach me a lesson. It was dehumanising; another time when all control was out of my hands and the balance of power was against me.

In the end they gave me an episiotomy – cutting me open with an incision that sounded like my mother's old kitchen scissors cutting bacon rind. I don't remember being asked – just told. There had been no mention of that at the antenatal classes or on the birth plan.

I left the labour room feeling like I had been assaulted. I was sewn up, traumatised, depressed, distanced from the world and from myself, and with a deep and abiding anger at the labour ward staff.

I phoned a friend but did not have the words to describe how I felt. With relief she said, 'You sound exactly the same!' But I was not the same; I had crossed into new and frightening territory.

Because Nina was born three weeks early, Cello had to go to work for a few hours before I'd had a chance to get cleaned up. He came back with a copy of that day's *Scotland on Sunday* newspaper with the headline 'England win with a touch of bad grace'. Apparently somewhere out in the real world the England rugby team had won the Grand Slam. It was hard to imagine that outside this alien, other-worldly maternity ward where I was still covered in blood and sweat from giving birth, woozy from lack of sleep, and utterly overwhelmed by the responsibility of a new baby, there were those who still cared about sporting fixtures and winning trophies. I put the newspaper aside, left the baby with Cello, and went for a bath.

On the ward over the next few days, I had no sleep, aches all over my body and a baby who was struggling to feed. Nothing seemed real; I was not me any more – I was a mother who was already failing despite having been in the role for only a few hours.

There were strict rules forbidding you to walk about with your baby, which must be pushed around in a wheel-along plastic cot. On the fourth or fifth night I grabbed her from her plastic cot and set off in my nightie with bare feet out of the ward. I roamed blindly along 120-year-old hospital corridors, like some Victorian ghost, gripping Nina, no idea where I was going.

Anywhere was better than there.

I saw the payphone but had no money, so the only number I could ring was the freephone number for *The Scotsman* news-paper where Cello worked as a reporter – a number for people with publishable stories to contact a journalist. Holding tightly to Nina, I dialled it. Cello was not on late shift, so was not in the *Scotsman* building. I begged the baffled late-night telephone operator: *Phone Cello, tell him I need to come home.*

As I clung to the phone, a midwife walked past; she was East Asian with a soft face and a gentle voice. 'Where are you going?' Her concern made me start to cry. She took my baby from me and said she would care for her until morning in the nursery. She led me back to my bed, tucked me in and drew the curtains.

I never knew her name, but I remember her kindness clearly.

A week later, I left hospital feeling I didn't have the right to complain because of course childbirth was hard, it was the same for every woman; nothing else mattered because I had a healthy baby. I joined what felt like a conspiracy of silence; childbirth was fine, the baby was fine, I was fine.

Fourteen

Now, here I was again, trapped alone and powerless in hospital, this time on a cancer ward.

Lunchtime came and went, and I continued to wait.

It was three hours since the wire had been inserted, and the local anaesthetic was wearing off. Not only that, but the wire was fighting against the dressing and was popping out of one side.

Two of the other ladies returned from surgery and the first, a woman who had had her entire breast removed and reconstructed, asked for a ham sandwich and a cup of tea.

'We used to have a toaster,' said the nurse apologetically, 'but they took it away. Health and safety.'

At 2.30pm a nurse gave me a last check: name and date of birth? Forms signed? Anti-embolism stockings on? Make-up and nail varnish removed? All jewellery removed? I panicked, remembering a diamante stud in the cartilage in my upper ear – I had no idea how to get it out. Again, that disconcerting feeling of being unprepared, in control of nothing. They covered it with an Elastoplast like in a school PE lesson.

I was wheeled towards the operating theatre into an ante-room full of activity: people putting things away, getting things out, flicking through papers on clipboards, talking over me. There were double doors at my feet – the doors the patient never sees beyond. 'Who's in there?' I asked. The surgeon, the nurse and the orderly, explained a chatty nurse, who showed me her tattoo and modelled two scrub caps with natty patterns. Afterwards I had no recollection of what her tattoo was or whether her scrub caps were natty or not, but I clearly remembered her friendliness.

The anaesthetist put a drip into the back of my hand and began to administer the anaesthetic. There was an agonising burning.

'Stop it!' I panicked, trying to shake the line away, half rising off the bed. 'Stop it!'

And that was the last I knew.

'Hello, Catherine, it's all over.' A nurse loomed over me as I had the sensation of being dredged from the bottom of the sea. I closed my eyes and wished her away.

After what could have been five minutes or two hours, I was wheeled from the recovery room back to the ward, where all of the other women were propped up in bed chatting.

I was out of sync again.

There was no sense of relief, only exhaustion, and a fear of moving.

I lay in bed listening to that morning's surgeon doing his rounds, visiting all of the other women in the ward. This surgeon had a masterful bedside manner. He was Northern English with a booming voice. Curtains were drawn around each bed as he visited, but the privacy was only token – the rest of the ward could hear every word he said as well as the women's murmured replies.

He reassured one woman, 'It was pre-cancerous, you've not got cancer or anything...' and I wished someone would say that to me. He disappeared behind the next curtain: 'I took tissue from this area ... we'll have to see when the swelling goes down ... if we aren't satisfied, we can book you in for another procedure ... but don't worry ... I'll see you in clinic!'

He came to the lady in the next bed and the curtain was swept closed with a rattling flourish. He asked if she was comfortable, and she explained where it hurt. The next minute he burst from behind the curtain, dashed away and came back moments later brandishing a soft white bra. 'Try this!' he said, vanishing back behind the curtain.

I wanted this man to come and talk to me – despite him having nothing to do with my care. With his Northern English accent, he even spoke my language. I longed for some of his warmth, energy and reassurance. Merely listening to him raised my confidence and made me shuffle up a bit in the bed. But, of course, once he had chatted with his own patients, he disappeared.

A little later my own surgeon appeared at my bedside dressed in green scrubs, including the cap. He explained that he had taken the cancerous tumour away along with some extra healthy tissue all around. He said he would see me in three weeks in his clinic when the results of the pathology would be back. Then he began to leave. As he reached the end of the bed, he looked over his shoulder: 'Oh and don't drive straight away,' then he shrugged. '... or ask your insurance.' And with that he was gone.

I don't remember speaking a word.

Later I related this to the friend who had told me how charming my surgeon was and how she always put her best bra on for his consultations.

'Ooooh, scrubs!' she said, widening her eyes. 'I'd like to have seen *that*.'

I also told a doctor friend about it and he sympathised with the surgeon: 'Think how *boring* his job is, doing the same thing every day', and I was affronted at the implication that operating on my body would be boring.

As I sat in my hospital bed, it seemed odd to have mixed feelings about someone who had just saved my life.

Doctors are powerful people. They hold all the cards. I have known that since I shoved a plastic jewel up my nose aged four and the doctor who got it out with tweezers dropped it clanking into a kidney dish and refused to give it back. My sister and I had been playing 'Cows and Bulls' – I was the bull so *naturally* I had needed a ring in my nose. I burned with impotent fury at the green jewel lost in the kidney-shaped dish, as my mother laughed.

But I said nothing; I had been voiceless then and I was voiceless now.

After a few hours, when I had the strength to walk to the bathroom, I got rid of the hospital gown and rooted out the old-lady non-underwired bra from my bag. I fastened it gingerly, taking care not to disturb the big dressing. My face was grey in the mirror, but at least it wasn't blue. As I headed back to bed, the world began to sink under my feet. The nurse was sitting in my chair reading out a list of instructions for when I got home. 'Keep your dressing on for ten to fourteen days. No spray deodorants. No shaving under the arm. No lifting anything heavier than a full kettle for six weeks...' She looked up, as my knees buckled. 'Ooh, she's having a whitey!'

I had been away from home for only twelve hours, but I was as homesick as if I had been travelling the far reaches of the planet for twelve months.

I was surprised to find that the 'old lady' bra I had so resented felt like my best friend, holding me close and keeping me safe. My black lacy underwired bras were instantly redundant: uncomfortable and archaic.

I had jumped a generation and joined my daughters, who would never dream of wearing uncomfortable underwear, who gave no thought to 'uplift' and were not embarrassed by the shape of a nipple.

My great-grandmother's generation had been strapped into corsets, laced right up the back to create a 'wasp' waist – one advert making the unlikely claim: *Every breath a free one, every move an easy one.* My grandmother's generation struggled into panty girdles with *layers of elastic and satin, bones, hooks-and-eyes, zippers and sometimes straps and buckles,* to flatten the stomach, smooth the bottom and hold their stockings up. My mother's generation – the ones who were not burning their bras (and *none* was apparently burning their bras within a million miles of me) – had *cross-your-heart* bras, robust elastic engineering that promised to *lift and separate* to make you *shapelier and prettier.*

At least my mother's generation were done with suspenders and stockings and could happily embrace American Tan nylons. However, they (and I) stuck with petticoats for some time; shiny, lace-edged slips to stop dresses clinging or being transparent – all the better to be modest. How we goggled at nineteen-year-old Lady Diana Spencer in 1980, photographed inadvertently in a see-through skirt, and who allegedly said: *I don't want to be known as the girlfriend who had no petticoat.*

Each generation had been controlled, trussed up, trapped, confined and shaped in different ways to fulfil the 'ideal' woman's body of the time and each generation must have looked back with relief that they were not subject to the same undergarments as their mothers.

Likewise, I had thought I was fortunate because underwear, when I was in my twenties, was colourful and did not look like medical apparatus.

But in fact, I had a troubled history with bras.

At school some of the boys would try to guess my bra size: 32B? 34C? Showing their 'sophistication' by knowing that bras and breasts had official sizes at all.

Thing is, I did not have a bra size, not one I knew anyway; I wore hand-me-downs, bras that didn't fit, leftover bras drifting around the back of the airing cupboard, abandoned bras with no elastic left, bras with knots tied in the straps to try to make them comfortable.

One day at high school I decided to ask to leave the top set in Maths. I didn't like Maths and it was making me miserable – but I was unable to put my hand up in class in case my ill-fitting bra shot up around my neck. I ended up staying in the top set and hating A-Level Maths rather than studying a subject I liked. I left school at eighteen with poor results. For the want of some bra elastic, my education was lost (at least for a time).

When I had the money to buy my own bras, I squeezed into the smallest size possible. To be a 36C was acceptable – anything bigger would be embarrassing, too blowsy. What exactly was blowsy? My *Oxford Paperback Dictionary* said it was 'red-faced and coarse-looking', but I knew there was a subtext – something to do with big breasts and low-cut tops, possibly on a barmaid.

I was eventually fitted properly for a bra in my twenties, by a no-nonsense woman in a posh 'ladieswear' shop, where I discovered I was a 34F.

This was odd because being a 36C had become part of my identity (like when a friend informed me that my birthday was 'on the cusp' so I was *actually* a Libra, not a Scorpio). Anyway, officially being a 34F didn't make much difference because chain stores did not stock that size then. On the odd occasion I could afford to buy one in a fancy shop, it looked vast and startling and there was always a risk that boyfriends would entertain themselves by wearing it like a hat. *Your tits are the same size as my head!*

Bras were expensive, even from ordinary shops, and must be worn until they were 'done', which usually meant until the underwire broke free and unknown to you poked through your jumper like an antenna, while you were out shopping.

I had always believed that cleavage was 'common' – too Bet Lynch – maybe it was being brought up by the 'lift-and-separate' generation, but surely breasts should never meet in public to create a deep and vulgar valley?

However, when I was thirty, everyone was suddenly wearing 'push-up' bras, in particular, Wonderbras, with their controversial 'Hello Boys!' traffic-stopping billboards showing a supermodel's cleavage. It was said that push-up bras made your breasts 'pneumatic', which was a puzzle – the *Oxford English Dictionary* definition: *pneumatic: filled with or operated by compressed air*.

So with my push-ups bras, not only was I wearing uncomfortable underwire, with unwanted padding, but a bra that made me feel I was in danger of spilling out all over the table.

In the 1990s and 2000s, many different types of bra became necessary: half-cup 'balcony' bras for low-cut tops; super-smooth 'T-shirt' bras to banish and deny the very existence of the nipple; sports bras; bras with see-through straps; bras with straps that could be fixed in any number of ways; bras with no straps at all; plus, an array of basques and body-forming Spanx knickers, which were not a million miles away from what my grandmother wore.

The shops were full of 'matching sets' – bra and knickers in lace, silk, satin, in flowery designs, bold colours, and all things bright and beautiful. This was a far cry from my childhood, when my sewing-mad mother bought one pair of nice knickers then unpicked them and used the bits as a pattern to make lots more pairs in pale pink.

As an adult, comfort was never a priority, nor usually a consideration. For years I wore G-strings to avoid the dreaded VPL – visible panty line – which were not comfortable, but I considered the discomfort worth it.

One day I watched my Italian mother-in-law, who was helping to fold my laundry, as she encountered a G-string; she puzzled over it, stretching it in various directions, then went to fetch her reading glasses so she could more closely examine this mysterious item.

But despite all of the underwear bought, an event to be savoured every day was the moment I got home from work and could take off my bra. The blessed relief, the blissful release; yet I never thought, should it be this way? Should my underwear be painful?

Now here I was post-cancer op, back home, nervous of moving, heart cushion clutched to my wound and so grateful for my comfortable bra.

I contacted the woman who made the healing cushion to thank her and wrote about the cushion on Facebook, which prompted an online discussion about how acts of kindness such as this were rarely extended to mental health hospitals. I was taken aback and for a moment took the remark personally (did they *resent* me getting *a cushion*), until, on reflection, I realised they had a point: breast cancer came with the privilege of sympathy.

Gifts arrived: flowers in vases, flowers flat-packed to fit through the letterbox, flowers with chocolates, flowers with books, virtual flowers, notebooks, toiletries, theatre tickets.

I am bad at receiving gifts. I have always found it a mortifying performance: unwrapping the present as the giver watches, finding the right words, making the right facial expressions. The whole experience embarrasses me. But this was different; these gifts meant a lot because they formed a barrier between me and reality. I had so many spectacular flower arrangements that 'refreshing the flowers' became a daily task.

One morning, as I refilled a vase, I got an inkling as to why there is such a thing as Munchausen syndrome: a mental illness that causes people to feign ill-health to gain attention and sympathy. For a moment, being the recipient of so much care, so much goodwill, so many flowers, seemed heady, almost exciting. I felt valued, approved of, accepted, as though I had done something special, as though I had *achieved* something.

Fourteen

It was surprising what cancer was teaching me about myself.

My hairdresser, Linden, washed my hair to help me protect my wound. She gave me coffee and a head massage and refused payment.

Acts of kindness like that seemed profound.

I had nineteen days to wait to find out whether the cancer had spread into the lymph nodes. Had it spread beyond the lymph nodes? Were cancer cells already floating about in my body waiting to take root elsewhere?

The days yawned ahead, leaving me in a terrible half-life.

Someone said, 'Two weeks on Tuesday – that's no time.'

And I wanted to slap them.

I wanted to fast-forward and not live through those days, but at the same time, I didn't want to waste a moment. I became obsessed with trying to 'bank' time, squirrelling it away, wanting to preserve moments in aspic, to hold them and never let them go; in effect, to stop time.

I decided to do something new every day, something small, tiny but memorable.

I took different routes around the city; turning right rather than left; exploring closes I had previously bypassed; using different shops and cafés. I ate pork gyoza dumplings, chicken yakisoba, baba ganoush, fattoush and kubbeh. I made Massaman curry and drank Negronis, Appletinis and plum wine. I wore silver and gold eyeshadow and tried not to look like I'd lost my heart to a starship trooper. I attended my first boxing match and went to Ladbrokes and lost a bet on 'Posh Trish' in the 4.50 at Cheltenham. I read poetry by Emily Dickinson, lyrics by Patti Smith and listened to T. S. Eliot reading 'The Waste Land' as I folded the washing. I watched *A Clockwork Orange* and random channels on the television, until one of them tried to sell me a royal commemorative coin for fifty quid. I planted indoor hyacinths. I listened to Purcell and Bartok on my mother's old vinyl records and I bathed in water gritty with Himalayan salt.

By this route of small new things, I ventured through those fearful days.

Fifteen

I was given strong painkillers after the operation, but the pain did not compare with the aftermath of giving birth and of breastfeeding.

When Nina was born, I had pulled the curtains around my hospital bed and hid. My body ached all over, I was nauseous with exhaustion and in despair that she would not feed. What was wrong with us? The other mothers chatted and padded around in slippers and prepared to go home.

'We need to get baby feeding before you go home,' declared the nurse, grasping my right breast as though it did not belong to me and thrusting it into the baby's face. 'Nose to nipple!' she instructed, 'nose to nipple!' But I didn't have enough hands to juggle breasts, nipples and baby. Sweat trickled down my back in the overheated ward.

The nurse shook her head: 'Well, they do say that bad babies make good toddlers.'

Nina is autistic, which obviously we didn't know then. Was that why she couldn't or wouldn't breastfeed? Did the smothering closeness of breastfeeding make her panic and fight? Who knows?

Except everyone thought they did.

Lean her this way ... move her that way ... try pinching here ... don't give up yet ... it's the best ... the cheapest ... the safest ... the most natural ... most convenient ... most moral choice there is ...

You've given up? Oh, what a shame ... I bet I could have got that baby to breastfeed ... it was probably about to start working ... If only you'd tried a bit harder ... for a bit longer.

I stayed in hospital a week, then went home in tears and agony for another fortnight as my first-born baby screamed for food but refused to latch on.

Throughout antenatal classes I had been bombarded with advice to breastfeed and given dire warnings about not doing so.

A bottle-fed baby is more likely to develop type 1 diabetes, to become obese, to get ear infections, diarrhoea, asthma, pneumonia....

Breast milk had been glibly described as: *available on tap! Always handy! Always ready! Always the right temperature – and free!* Warnings were given NOT to give your baby a bottle because a baby that so much as tasted milk from a bottle would not go back to breastfeeding.

As tension reached unbearable levels, my mother-in-law suggested a little bottle ... just a *little* bottle, may help, but I refused, half-hysterical: 'They've said giving a bottle will *spoil everything...*'

One dark and desperate evening I banged on the plate-glass door of Boots the Chemist, sobbing, moments after they shut for the night. The manageress, inside with a bunch of keys, hesitated at the sight of my tear-streaked face. I saw her expression – the desire to go home wrestling with the sight of my distress – and then she retraced her steps to unlock the door.

I begged for a packet of nipple shields.

They didn't help.

The next day I was still bleeding and crying, and my baby was crying and vomiting bloody milk. The counsellor from a breastfeeding charity, who had arrived from one of the posh houses up the road in response to my pleas for help, witnessed this as she perched on the end of my bed. She adjusted the kirby grip in her grey bob, dragged her home-knitted cardigan around her vast bosom and said, 'Maybe the odd bottle wouldn't hurt.'

So, I called it a day with the breastfeeding. It was only then that I realised caring for my newborn daughter did not have to be a horrendous, stressful, crying, agonising battle.

But the guilt lingered. Despite carrying and delivering a lovely baby, the shame of failure lingered.

After my second daughter, Lara, was born, the guilt about failing to breastfeed the first time remained strong.

The second time was as agonising as the first time, but at least this baby could breastfeed. I managed it for six months. The pain was extreme for the first few weeks, even with cold cabbage leaves stuck inside my bra to cool and soothe.

One day Cello begged me to stop and use a bottle as I fed the baby with tears running down my face. I refused; I could not fail again. I expressed milk, for an emergency supply, using a hand-held pump not unlike my dad's milking machine on the farm.

On a visit 170 miles away back to my childhood dairy farm, I became ill – feverish, with one breast red-hot and sore to the touch. When I mentioned it to my mum, my dad overheard and knew it would be mastitis – inflammation of the breast – because sometimes his milk cows got it and it necessitated a visit from the vet. 'That needs sorting out,' he declared.

The emergency doctor came and examined me in the best living room of the farmhouse – the room normally used only at Christmas. The room in which I was born. As we both stood between the Dralon sofa and the antique rocking chair, surrounded by gilt mirrors and gold-rimmed tea sets from my grandparents' day, he gave me antibiotics, and advised me to keep feeding through the pain.

Twenty-one years after I last breastfed, as I was writing this, I saw a poster from a maternity hospital: *Did you know that a baby who is fed formula milk eats 30,000 more calories than a breastfed baby by 8 months of age. That is equivalent to 120 Mars Bars. Once a child becomes obese it is likely they will remain obese into adulthood.*

Anger flared and I realised how much resentment I still harboured about the bullying over breastfeeding. As a new mother, I had been wrung out physically and mentally and it had been impossible to make a sensible decision.

It reminded me again how hard it is in life to know when to say 'yes' (what James Joyce called the 'female word') and when to say 'no'.

Helen Mirren famously said that if she were to give advice to her younger self it would be to 'say fuck off more', and I say, 'oh yes'.

Sixteen

The prospect of chemotherapy terrified me.

I had watched both my parents go through chemo, which had looked painful, messy and debilitating. My mother suffered so many sessions it was hard to know if it was the cancer that killed her or the chemo. She died with numb finger-ends and a sore mouth because of the chemo; a large part of her final months was spent nauseous and weak because of the chemo. When I was fifteen, my father, who had got up to milk the cows every morning of my childhood, come hell or high water, without a day's sickness, was knocked off his feet and into bed retching into a bucket because of his treatment for bone cancer.

It also made both of my parents lose their hair. My mother went from the traditional silver 'Queen Elizabeth' perm through a bald bandana stage to an eventual funky pixie cut. My father went from a Bobby Charlton comb-over through shiny baldness to short, wavy grey.

I was frightened of losing my hair.

Hair loss was punishment. I had read about the shearing of French women accused of Nazi collaboration to diminish and desexualise; the shaving, tarring and feathering of women who had fraternised with the enemy during the troubles in Northern Ireland, to humiliate and torture.

Having long dark hair was part of being me. I was one of three sisters all with long dark hair, which we considered a family trademark. In the eighties, people said we looked like Kate Bush, Chrissie Hynde and Cher.

As a child, I ate my bread crusts because Grandma said eating crusts would make my hair curl. The darker the crust, the curlier the hair; it made sense to me. Family photos show me at four years old with a pudding-bowl 'Beatles' cut, ten years later with a pudding-bowl 'Purdey' cut and all the years in between with it straight-as-a-die with a ribbon on top.

My mother loved gadgets and invested in an 'Original Comet' – a comb with an inbuilt razor blade to 'cut, trim, groom and remove'. Apparently anyone could now do a professional haircut.

The reality was that it tugged and slashed and the results were what you would realistically expect of a razor blade wedged in a comb. It was abandoned after a single hair-cutting session. Fifty years later, twelve years after my mother's death, I discovered 'The Original Comet Safety Haircutter, Patent Pending' in the bottom of her ottoman still with lengths of shiny brown hair stuck in its teeth.

Through the years I have attempted Farrah Fawcett flick-ups, Diana side-swipes, a long bob, a short bob, a page-boy, a feather cut – it has even verged on a mullet. It has been permed, straightened, crimped, dyed raven black and auburn, bleached and streaked. In the eighties I was a dab hand with the heated rollers and the curling tongs, every single morning. On my wedding day it was wrenched into a French roll with cream roses fixed so firmly it took an hour to get the pins out.

Like my good health, I have taken my hair for granted.

Except when I got alopecia.

Twice, at times of stress, I have discovered perfect bald circles on my scalp, each a little bigger than a 10-pence piece. The first time was the day I discovered my mother's cancer was terminal. The contrast between the baby-pink soft bald patches and the thick dark hair was shocking, almost obscene, but I tied my hair up every day to hide the bald patch and chose not to panic.

Someone joked that I should colour my circle of bare scalp with boot polish because that was how Victorian men hid a bald patch and I laughed, but it felt like a punch. I did not consult a doctor, because I knew there was no treatment. If it grew back, it grew back; if it all fell out, it all fell out.

Slowly baby wisps appeared, and it grew back.

But if I needed chemo, I knew I would not hang on to it and hope for the best. It would be shorn immediately. I did not want it falling out in the shower, or to find handfuls clinging around the house or blowing like tumbleweed across the carpet. I would not drag it from the plughole entangled with my daughter's blue-dyed hair or find it beside me on the pillow when I woke up.

My mother spent years complaining that her three long-haired daughters ruined her hoovers, as though we shed hair on purpose. I would not be cutting my lost hair off my hoover brushes.

I Googled 'pixie cut' and 'Jamie Lee Curtis'. I Googled 'chemo hats'. I discovered such things as 'scarf pads', 'scarf grips' and 'false fringes' that create an illusion of a full head of hair.

I read celebrity accounts of chemotherapy written with the stated aim of reassuring other women. They did not reassure me. They terrified me. I vowed I would never wear the terrible-sounding 'cold cap' – a tight-fitting hat worn during the infusion of chemo drugs to cool the scalp and help prevent hair loss. This thing sounded like torture, causing ice-cream headaches and chattering teeth. The cap contained gel cooled to a temperature of between -15° and -40° Fahrenheit and had to be worn before, during and after each treatment.

No. I would rather go bald.

I would buy enormous earrings. I would wear turbans. I would be early Carole Lombard and late Elizabeth Taylor. I would channel Sophia Loren on the cover of *Vogue*. I would fasten brooches to my turbans and festoon them in pearls and feathers. I would buy them in leopard print. I would wear beanies – fleecy ones and knitted ones and ones with enormous pom-poms on top. I would wear scarves in satin and silk and silver and paisley. I would knot the scarves at the back, at the front or on the top, channelling Grace Kelly, Jackie O or Rosie the Riveter with her bulging muscles. I would wear false eyelashes and have my eyebrows tattooed back on. I would learn to tie a head wrap. I would rock a cloche. I would buy wigs in punky pink and blue and borrow my daughter's waist-length rusty-red wig. I would wear the Ruby Woo lipstick regardless, and choose jewellery that was bigger and bigger, brighter and brighter.

If necessary, I would invent a whole new me.

But I was still terrified of losing my hair.

Of course, it would not only be the hair on my head I would lose – and this could have been the sole upside of chemotherapy. Leg hair had been a bane since puberty. Shaving, waxing, depilating, epilating, I had had a lifelong fight with hair-removal methods that didn't work: the ingrowing hairs and the pain of epilating; the cost and the forest of hair required for waxing; the stink of the chemicals when depilating; the cuts, the bleeding ankle divots, the shin slices and the stubble of shaving. When my nephew was a toddler and knew very few words, he accidentally brushed his hand across my leg and said, 'Ooh, sharp!'

Trying to have smooth legs was expensive and *so time-consuming* – I wonder how many hours I have spent shaving my legs? Besides, it was inconvenient; you could guarantee the day you hadn't shaved would be the day the sun came out, and stubbly legs were yet another thing to be self-conscious about when you went for smear tests.

I remember being fascinated by the dark hairs squashed under American Tan tights as I hid under dinner tables as a child in the seventies, but as I grew up, I realised that dark body hair on a woman was taboo, shameful, unacceptable.

Things were no different for my daughters. In 2017, when Nina decided to stop shaving and went out with leg hair, my friend Carole remarked, 'Well done, Nina! That takes balls.' And it did; in the same year, model Arvida Byström got rape threats for appearing in the Adidas Superstar campaign with unshaven legs.

And it wasn't just leg hair. Online porn had apparently made *any* body hair unacceptable to my daughters' generation – many of whom have apparently had their pubic hair permanently removed.

Discussing this, Lara looked astounded: 'What? In the eighties you had a full bush?!'

Cello and I looked at each other.

'Er … yes.'

Eventually, the year before the cancer diagnosis, I finally solved this perennial problem by having all of my leg hair lasered off.

I lay on the treatment bed, every few weeks for several months, as me and the therapist, wearing matching goggles, discussed the preparations for her daughter's wedding – the exact shade of pink for the bridesmaid dresses, the canapes, the singing butlers – and she rubbed ultrasound gel all over my legs then moved the laser up and down as concentrated light beams destroyed my hair follicles. It cost hundreds of pounds and felt like hot little insect bites, but it was worth every penny and every moment of discomfort to never have to think about leg hair ever again.

Seventeen

'You *are* making light of it,' a friend said.

In truth, I did not know how I was going to survive more waiting to discover the exact cancer treatment I would need.

I sought out animal rescue stories: dogs dug out of wells, plucked from swollen rivers and brought home from war zones. Cats pulled out of drains and abandoned buildings, discovered in knotted sacks and locked sheds.

I needed a happy ending.

I found myself staring for long minutes at a film of nothing but a dog asleep on a hammock.

I was overcome by stark, disabling terror that caused a tightening at the top of my stomach, making my breathing shallow. At any moment I would start gasping. A twisting lower in my stomach made me feel sick. I wasn't part of the normal world. I was alone in my own prison.

To escape, even if only for a while, I went to the cinema next door.

It was a twelve-screen multiplex, part of a big chain, not one of the quirky independent cinemas — with leather sofas, art deco coffee bars or prosecco by the bottle — that I, like a snob, would have preferred to live beside. No, this was the Vue and it was 200 steps from my front door and only £5.99 a film.

The obsession with escaping into films began a few days after my operation. I was alone as the 6 o'clock news came on and was suddenly overwhelmed by the encroaching darkness. Watching day turn to dusk made the cinema irresistible. I grabbed my money and my heart-shaped cushion and went, not caring what was showing.

In the cinema, I hugged the cushion to protect and dampen the pain under my arm and gazed at the screen mesmerised.

This was unusual. I had always preferred to get my stories from books. But now I couldn't concentrate on books unless they were about cancer. I had tried to read other stuff, but it didn't seem important. Learning about cancer was paramount.

But films were different.

I was not brought up in a film-watching family. My mother tried it once. She took my best friend, Alex, and me to the cinema in 1977, when we were fourteen, to see *Annie Hall*. She said she had read it was a masterpiece, although I can't imagine where because she only read the *Daily Express*, and *Annie Hall* was a film about sex. It was supposed to be a comedy, but I don't remember any of us laughing. All I recall was a reference to an orgasm and my mother rolling her eyes with her entire body. The journey home was quiet and as my mother dropped Alex off she said to Alex's mum, 'Well, I don't know what *that* was all about.'

Not long afterwards, my mother, my little sister Tricia and I went on holiday to a B&B in London. It was 1978, the week the film *Grease* was released. My mother had learned her lesson; she would not be sitting through another film about nothing but sex. Tricia and I watched John Travolta and Olivia Newton-John on two consecutive nights and *Grease* was indeed the word, the word that we heard, and it *did* have groove and it *did* have meaning. Meanwhile, my mother sat alone in the screen next door watching *Hercule Poirot* and *Grizzly Adams*.

Growing up in the country ten miles from the nearest cinema – the ABC in Lancaster – meant films passed me by. In 1966 I was just too young for *The Sound of Music* and for a fortnight afterwards had to put up with big sister Elizabeth singing 'I am sixteen going on seventeen…'. In 1977 I was just too young for *Saturday Night Fever* and for the next fortnight had to put up with Elizabeth singing 'J-J-J-Jive Talkin''. I did not catch up with

Star Wars for forty years, by which time not having seen it had become a claim to fame.

In 1979 I went to watch Roger Moore in *Moonraker* with my friend, Carole. We sat on the bus in our matching anoraks and silver-rimmed specs. Somehow, I broke my glasses on the way, so Carole shared hers and we saw half the film each. I have still never seen an entire James Bond film.

My first boyfriend took me to the ABC to see Jack Nicholson in *The Postman Always Rings Twice*, only to discover it had stopped showing and the few remaining seats in the cinema were for *Caligula*. After watching unsimulated hardcore porn scenes featuring Playboy Bunnies, set in ancient Rome, the lights came up and I realised I was sitting beside my old maths teacher.

All in all, the cinema was not an obvious place for me to seek sanctuary in those nineteen days of waiting. But a sanctuary it became.

I went back many times during that interminable time; the screen was so BIG, it helped drown out the enormity of what was happening in the real world. It was important I was alone; I wanted to feel uncoupled from reality. It was me and the screen, the screen and me. I willingly handed over responsibility for the next two hours.

It became a ritual: the purchase of a £1 bag of Revels at Tesco across the road; the queue for the ticket; the walk along the artificially lit, popcorn-strewn carpet past the electronic adverts and through the heavy doors.

It was the whump of the soundproofed doors closing behind me that separated me from real life. Now I was sealed in another place that could be anywhere.

This is not a cinema, it said on screen, in a Magrittian touch. *This is a racetrack. This is a festival. This is a legendary opera house. This is not a cinema.*

I ate the Revels as soon as the lights went down; I had no interest in deferring gratification. Orange, Malteser, Malteser, orange, toffee, chocolate penny. The sickly-sweet flavours finished before the opening credits rolled.

So few people were there at these odd hours during the week, it felt like my own cinema, my own space, and if there was the rustle of a popcorn bucket or the rattle of a sweet packet, I was taken aback.

I loved the dimming of the lights and the deep booming voice: *Boo! Makes you feel alive, doesn't it? A little scare ... A little darkness...*

I loved the trailers: *It's the tale of a journey: a journey we take to prove ourselves. It's about courage...* Which trailer was that? It could have been any of them, or all of them.

Then the plug for MediCinema, a charity providing films in hospital to help children through difficult times. I realised I had created my own MediCinema here at the Vue – and it was making me feel better, if only for a couple of hours at a time.

Get Ready. Take your seat. Switch off from the outside world.

And I did, again and again.

Handing over power was an enormous relief, not like the handing over of power in a hospital, which was exposing and made me vulnerable and anxious; with this handing over of power, I felt safe and protected.

I didn't choose by genre, or indeed any other category; I wanted a film to fill my head and, like a centrifugal force, push cancer to the edges, to enable me to leave this reality and enter a different one. When the overthinking became unbearable, the immensity of the cinema gave my brain a reboot; it switched it off and switched it on again. But it had to be the cinema – when I got DVDs from the library to watch at home they didn't work. I was not hermetically sealed from the world sitting on the sofa; a television screen was just too small to help.

The cinema was about watching characters overcoming something bigger than themselves, watching characters battling their demons and winning.

Whether it was dynasties fighting dynasties, parents fighting children, criminals fighting the law, individuals overcoming addiction, betrayal, poverty or prejudice, in this world or the next, today, yesterday or tomorrow, I wanted to watch characters thinking they were trapped but then finding a way out, characters struggling then emerging triumphant, characters dealing with fear.

When in an opening line of *Lady Bird*, Saoirse Ronan said, 'I wish I could *live* through something', she took me back to my fourteen-year-old self, lying on the back lawn of our farmhouse watching planes flying to and from Manchester Airport, when I had longed to escape and for something, *anything*, to happen; surely *any* drama was better than none.

You must be careful what you wish for.

The philosopher Ludwig Wittgenstein used to dash to the cinema, after lecturing at Cambridge University, to sit in the front row munching a bun or a cold pork pie. He wanted his whole field of vision to be taken up by the screen and rarely took his eyes off it so he could free his mind from thoughts that tortured him.

Sitting in the Vue, I felt a kinship with this dead philosopher furiously munching on his cold pork pie, losing himself in another world, his face bathed in flickering light from the cinema screen.

Two weeks after the operation, I removed the dressing myself. I was told one of the breast cancer nurses would remove it if I wished, because, 'Some people think it will all burst open, but it won't.'

I held my breath and gently peeled it off. The scar was dark purple and about 8 cm long. There was only one scar – the cancer and the lymph nodes must have been removed from the same incision – I had expected two. The surgeon had cut precisely within the suntan line left by my bikini. I wondered if this was coincidence, but I was grateful.

The appointment to get my results on day twenty was in the afternoon. I had a hairdresser's appointment that morning, which had been in the diary for months. I decided to go and get my hair coloured despite knowing it may only be on my head for another week or two.

I listened to the supervisor advising my stylist on the subtleties of dye application: 'Give it fifteen minutes under heat rather than forty minutes without,' she picked up a strand, 'and try to lift these mid-tones.'

All this effort, at a considerable cost, was an act of defiance and bravado.

As I left, I put the hairdressers on standby. 'I'll be right back to get it cut off if needs be.' No problem, they said, they were ready if required. They smiled and waved, and I waved back, giving them a thumbs-up through the window. I looked braver than I felt, or maybe not, maybe the terror was writ large across my face.

The waiting room in the Breast Unit was busy but at least a busy waiting room is better than a fear-amplifying quiet waiting room. I checked my watch repeatedly. I thought motherhood had taught me patience, but motherhood had nothing on cancer.

At last my consultant surgeon appeared at the door, reading my notes and calling my name. This was the surgeon I had seen so little of at the time of the operation.

I braced myself and followed him into his room, but before Cello and I had time to sit down he said, 'It's all good news. The lymph nodes are clear. There will be no chemotherapy.'

I was stunned. Later I was grateful he had not kept us waiting even for another minute, and I forgave him any perceived slights from the day of the op, but at that moment I was stunned. I had expected the worst; every bit of me was poised for bad news.

I had a notebook on my lap with questions jotted down. It was a ridiculous tiny notebook with a holographic cover that I had won in a cracker. What possessed me to write the questions in there? I could not focus on the words.

He asked how I was, and I said my underarm felt as though it had been scoured with a wire brush.

'Oh, yes, because that's *exactly* what we have done,' he joked, so I shut up.

He told me I would need radiotherapy to kill any remaining cancer cells in the breast, and that he had set up an appointment for me in two days to get it arranged. The radiotherapy would start in the next fortnight – not too soon after the surgery, he said, so 'everything doesn't collapse,' adding hurriedly, when he saw the stricken look on my face, 'not that it will'.

He explained that because my cancer had tested positive for oestrogen receptors, I would be on the anti-oestrogen drug tamoxifen for ten years. He printed a prescription for me to take to the hospital pharmacy, muttering something about side effects, as he tapped on his keyboard.

What did he mean? What side effects? How bad?

I was mute.

I deciphered a word in my shiny cracker notebook. It said: *Why?* And I asked, 'Why did I get this?'

He grimaced to indicate there was no straightforward answer, then said, 'Statistically speaking – (and he enunciated each syllable) *Stat-is-tic-ally speak-ing* – it was the HRT that caused it, but we could never prove it.'

I learned later there is a name for this sort of thing: iatrogenic illness. An illness caused by medical intervention, because I believed he was right; it was the HRT.

'Oh, I suppose I'd better have a look,' he said.

He asked me to go behind the curtain and remove my upper clothing and he opened the door to the corridor and shouted for a nurse to come in. I perched on the side of the bed as he looked at the scar on my right breast. The nurse flew in from the corridor, dodging round the curtain, still laughing at some joke from outside. 'That scar's looking good,' he muttered, more to himself then to me. The nurse was still chuckling.

I felt diminished; nothing but a scar.

Having psyched myself up for the worst, I was surprised to leave the consultant's office with an anti-climactic mix of numbness and shock. I felt punch-drunk.

As I waited for the tamoxifen at the hospital pharmacy, I bought a coffee from the WRVS stall and posted on Facebook: *No need for chemo and the radiotherapy should be done by Christmas. Bloody marvellous. Celebrating in the WRVS café…*

Marvellous? Celebrating? What whopping lies we tell on social media.

At home I reached to the top of the kitchen cabinet and found the pink pack of HRT that I couldn't bear to throw away two months ago when Lizzie the breast care nurse told me to stop taking it.

This was the drug that probably gave me cancer.

I fished out the information leaflet – a tissue-thin, multi-folded strip of paper that when straightened out was more than three feet long with tiny writing on both sides. As usual, there was a seemingly all-encompassing list of *Possible Side Effects*: ovarian cancer, cancer of the lining of the womb, blood clots, heart disease, stroke, but heading the list was 'breast cancer'. Halfway down the other side was a section: **Breast Cancer:** *Evidence suggests that taking combined oestrogen-progestogen and possibly also oestrogen-only HRT increases the risk of breast cancer. The extra risk depends on how long you take HRT. The additional risk becomes clear within a few years.*

There was a shaded box entitled **Compare**, which said: *Women aged 50 to 79 who are not taking HRT, on average 9 to 17 in 1,000 will be diagnosed with breast cancer over a 5-year period. For women aged 50 to 79 who are taking oestrogen-progestogen HRT over 5 years, there will be 13 to 23 cases in 1,000 users (ie an extra 4 to 6 cases).*

Advice was given to do regular breast checks and to take offered mammogram screening.

I had never read this leaflet before.

Who expects to be one of the *extra 4 to 6 cases* in one thousand? Who expects to be so unlucky? Clearly not me; especially as I was only forty-four when I started taking HRT, and yet it is obvious that *somebody* must be that unlucky.

And if not me, then who?

The hardest things in my life have always been because I live in a female body.

Two days later, I was back at the Western to organise my radiotherapy schedule.

I had assumed I would feel better now the threat of chemotherapy had gone, but instead I felt becalmed, frustrated and sunk in inertia. The worry about remaining cancer cells in my body made me unproductive. I couldn't write, and this lack of productivity increased my anxiety about wasted time – round and round it went in a downward spiral.

Time was at once a burden to be endured and something precious and tactile and beautiful, like silk, slipping through my fingers.

It was a Thursday, and I knew they were recording an episode of *Question Time* in the Scottish Parliament that evening. I had applied for a place but heard nothing. I decided to try my luck and phone the producers to ask instead. *Question Time* has been part of my life since I was a teenager watching Robin Day with my dad. This was to be one of David Dimbleby's final recordings.

As far as wanting to do something new every day, this was a good one.

Sitting in the Oncology waiting room, I phoned the producers and got an answer machine on which I left a message. Ten minutes later, the producer called back just as I heard, 'Catherine, can you come though now?'

I thrust the phone at Cello, asking him to talk to the producer and get me a ticket, and I went into the oncologist's room only to find Cello sitting down beside me having rung off. I knew it was ridiculous to be concentrating on tickets for *Question Time* when I was supposed to be talking to this doctor about cancer treatment, but it took a lot of resolve not to start a fight: 'Why did you ring off?! I wanted those tickets!'

The doctor explained I needed fifteen sessions of radiotherapy – one a day for three weeks.

Radiotherapy frightened me: it is carcinogenic; it seems contrary to use it to kill cancer. Would it do me more harm than good?

The doctor did nothing to assuage my fears. She ploughed through a list of things that could go wrong: in the short term, there could be skin burning and irritation and possibly blistering; fatigue was likely to set in that could last for months. Other side effects that could appear months or even years after treatment included: acute pneumonitis (inflammation of the lung); breast swelling, including shooting pains; breast changes, including becoming smaller and/or harder; chronic pneumonitis (hardening of a portion of the lung); rarely, bone thinning in the area of treatment; very rarely, heart complications could be triggered; swallowing problems and shoulder stiffness; nerve damage and lymphoedema.

There were so many 'coulds', 'maybes' and 'possiblies' it was hard to grasp. Would any of this happen? Would none of it happen? Did I have any choice?

What registered was the message: *This will damage you … this will make you feel terrible for months … sign here please.*

The doctor, sensing my fear, told me that after the surgery there was a one in three chance of the cancer returning, but after the radiation treatment there would be a one in twenty chance of it recurring. 'That's the figure you should keep in your mind,' she said.

I signed the form, but it felt wrong and unnatural to submit my body to radiation. Maybe all radiotherapy patients feel this way, or maybe it was a hangover from my mother's exploding mammogram story. I didn't know, but it highlighted the loss of control the cancer had brought with it.

I took it out on Cello and, when we left the consulting room, I snapped at him for putting the phone down on the *Question Time* producer. I stormed off to the hospital loo in a sulk. On the way home we went to Lidl. I could not read the labels on the jars of pesto and sun-dried tomatoes because my eyes were welling up. I bent low over the bottles and tins, pretending to study them, trying to hide the tears.

Cello suddenly appeared at my elbow holding out his mobile. While I had been in the hospital loo, he had texted the producers: *'My wife's being treated for cancer. She's upset because she wanted to come to tonight's show. I'm in trouble for cutting you off. Please give her a ticket.'*

The producer had phoned and was on the line. She didn't mention Cello's text or my cancer but asked how I had voted in the last election. I answered, trying not to sound like someone in Lidl weeping over jars of pickles in a fog of fear and despair. She was businesslike and it was good to be reminded that some women were leading lives unaffected by illness. Some women were thinking about politics and current affairs. Some women had television shows to produce and audiences to filter. It was good to feel her energy down the phone, to be involved, even for a minute or two, in something not connected with cancer.

She emailed two tickets.

Three hours later, we were at the Scottish Parliament, writing questions for the panel and being briefed by a dapper David Dimbleby in one of his trademark insect ties: 'This is your show,' he beamed at the assembled audience members. 'Get involved! Ask questions! If you agree with a panellist or contributor, clap! Enjoy yourselves!'

We watched the camera operators manoeuvring equipment around the famous *Question Time* semi-circular desk. A floor manager rehearsed us in clapping louder and louder, quieter and quieter, as he raised and lowered his arms. Five audience members were told their questions had been selected and were led off to practise. I was not one and was relieved; tonight, I was happy to be an observer.

I gazed around the Scottish Parliament debating chamber – a place I had seen on television but never expected to sit in – and I realised how much all this novelty was lifting my spirits. I thanked Cello for getting the tickets. 'Yeah, well,' he said, 'sometimes you have to ask for what you want.'

Eighteen

Edinburgh's Western General Hospital must be one of the ugliest hospitals, in fact one of the ugliest places.

It began life as a Victorian poorhouse in which the inmates were separated into different classes of accommodation. The men were split into 'very decent', 'decent', 'depraved' and 'boys', whereas the women were classed as 'decent', 'infirm', 'depraved', 'wasters', 'bastardy' and 'girls'. I know this because I became obsessed with finding out everything, however peripheral, about my cancer, even the history of the cancer hospital.

The Western had expanded in fits and starts over the years until it became an ugly tangle of buildings with a makeshift air, a hotch-potch of drab twentieth-century architecture huddled around the original confident Victorian poorhouse. There was a streaked-orange walkway leading to a sinister-looking chimney, which we drove under on each visit and which I learned was originally a state-of-the-art kidney transplant unit designed by renowned architect Peter Womersley. Perhaps it looked edgy and brutalist in the 1950s, with its concrete blocks and straight lines, but today it was the chemo ward and it just looked shabby and brutal. The very sight of it had a lowering effect and driving underneath felt like passing through a portal into the underworld.

Cello drove me to my 'measuring-up' appointment at the radiotherapy department – officially called 'treatment planning'. I clutched the letter with the radiotherapy schedule on it – a letter that entitled me to that most desirable of things: a guaranteed free parking spot in this chaotic, congested place.

I had not foreseen the day when one of my 'most desirable of things' would be a parking spot at the cancer hospital.

Here, men in hi-vis jackets and blue trousers waved their arms about, yelling, 'You can't stop here!' or 'Move along!' to hovering motorists, before bending down and asking through our car window, 'Have you got your letter?' I snatched it from my lap and held it up, two-handed, as though showing my passport at some far-off hostile border. The barrier slowly rose.

Radiotherapy is carried out every day for several weeks (except weekends and bank holidays) and if you live too far away to manage this, you live in the hospital grounds in a 'lodge' for the duration of the treatment. Fortunately, I lived only a twenty-minute drive away.

Today I was going to the building with the words 'Cancer Centre' in gold above sliding doors. I admired the chutzpah of the architect who chose gold lettering, which, although covered in a layer of dust, wouldn't have been out of place in a disco. I was also surprised by the bald, unadorned words 'Cancer Centre' – this place was not named after an eminent doctor or scientist, nor was it 'The Centre for Oncological Medicine', no, this was the straight-up Cancer Centre. I had not heard any medic use the word 'cancer' yet and I found myself nodding in approval at this ugly building.

Next to the sliding doors was a memorial bench: *In loving memory of John William MacDonald, Memories are a gift to treasure, Ours of you will last forever.* Each day as I entered the Cancer Centre, I looked out for someone smoking on this bench so I could sing the Editors song 'Smokers Outside the Hospital Doors' to myself and enjoy having seen a cliché in the wild, but it never happened. Instead, there were always elderly people rugged up waiting for hospital transport home. It was only later that I noticed the faded green diagonal lines painted in front of the doors with the worn-out ghosts-of-words *NO SMOKING ZONE.*

On that first day, Cello and I sat in a new waiting room down a long sloping corridor, because the radiotherapy machines must be located underground. A couple in their sixties were already waiting; it was obviously their first day, too. The man had a yellow pallor and the woman looked stunned. She perched on her seat and said, 'You look out of the window and the rest of the world is still carrying on, and you're stuck in a bubble...' We all nodded, and I instinctively glanced towards where the window should have been but was not because we were buried underground.

Up and down the corridor were illuminated signs saying *CONTROLLED AREA X-RAYS*, the words lit up in yellow on a black background alongside the symbol for radiation; the black circle surrounded by three black blades – a symbol designed to represent energy radiating from an atom but that reminded me of the top of one of my mother's cotton bobbins.

Did I find this hazard symbol so terrifying because I grew up during the Cold War? This black and yellow 'cotton bobbin' was as powerful a symbol as the skull and crossbones. In the seventies and eighties there was a constant fear of radiation: of atom bombs, nuclear warheads, intercontinental ballistic missiles, nuclear fallout, nuclear holocaust, nuclear apocalypse, radiation sickness, mushroom clouds, radioactive dust, Mutual Assured Destruction, President Regan's Star Wars, Ban the Bomb, nuclear meltdowns, *The China Syndrome* and Three-Mile Island. Blondie sang 'Atomic', Peter Gabriel sang about 'Games without Frontiers' and Frankie sang about 'Two Tribes' going to war.

At primary school I read the Marie Curie 'Great Scientists' Ladybird book, fascinated by Madame Curie in her austere Parisian garret with her glowing test tube, as the radium she'd discovered slowly killed her.

In high school English class, we read John Wyndham's *The Chrysalids*, with its post-apocalyptic landscape, mutants and outcasts, forever afterwards referring to any inhospitable place as 'The Badlands'.

We gave serious thought to what we would do if the four-minute warning sounded. This would apparently happen via sirens or the television or radio and was the length of time it took for an incoming nuclear missile to reach us and detonate.

What *would* we do in those four minutes? Who would we phone? What would we say? Where would we go? The 1984 BBC drama *Threads* showing Sheffield suffering a nuclear winter caused a stir. Then there was Chernobyl.

When my father had cancer in the early eighties, friends from abroad remarked that it was unsurprising he was ill – we lived near Windscale, what did we expect? Windscale, now known as Sellafield, was seventy-five miles further up the North-West coast. It was the site of the Windscale Fire of 1957 – the worst nuclear disaster in British history – when one of the nuclear reactors caught fire for three days and radioactive dust was spread across the UK and Europe. It was ranked at Level 5 out of a possible 7 on the International Nuclear Event Scale, and milk produced in the surrounding 500 square kilometres was diluted and thrown in the Irish Sea for a month afterwards.

And now here I was, sitting beneath a radiation warning sign waiting to be measured up so they could calculate exactly how much radiation to blast me with.

The measuring took place on a CT scanner in a big cold room. There was a tiny changing area in the corner with a blue semi-circular curtain to pull around me as I undressed. On the chair behind the curtain was a piece of crepe paper the size of a tea towel. 'That's a cover cloth for you,' the radiotherapist told me. I removed my top and clutching the 'cover cloth' emerged into the chill. The scanner had 'Philips' written on it – a name I had previously associated with hairdryers and screwdrivers.

Eighteen

There was another piece of crepe paper spread on the scanner bed and I lay on it as two or three young women technicians busied about. They got me into position with my arms stretched above my head in stirrups and told me to keep very still. They asked if I had any problem with keeping my arms above my head and I confidently told them that I had kept up my yoga throughout diagnosis and recovery from surgery and anyway I was double-jointed, so no, there would be no problem. A fortnight down the line I would remember this hubris and ask myself: haven't you learned *anything* about not taking your body for granted.

I asked if they would be looking for other tumours in my body when I went into the scanner and they hastily informed me this was a planning scan not a diagnostic scan. I felt foolish, but also disappointed. I would come for a scan every day of the week if they could reassure me I was cancer-free. My misunderstanding reinforced the fact that I was in the dark, really, about what was being done to me.

The scanner was a narrow bed that slid into a doughnut shape. I lay rigid, hardly daring to breathe, as the bed backed up into the machine. Before disappearing into the 'doughnut', the last thing I saw was a screen on the ceiling with an image of a blue, blue sky with fluffy white clouds. It reminded me of Southern Italy and was welcome in this austere room. I longed for an out-of-body experience – to be anywhere but here in this cold, cavernous room, on this enormous alienating machine.

One of the technicians put music on for me, so as I was swallowed by the machine I heard *Babe, there's something tragic about you...* and I didn't know whether to laugh or cry.

I couldn't tell if I was alone in the room because I wasn't allowed to move my head to look. The machine whirred and I concentrated on the music to pass the time and to stop myself panicking in this claustrophobic space.

'What was that music?' I asked when I emerged from the scanner shortly after and faces loomed above me.

'Hozier,' someone replied, 'and then the Saturdays, singing "Lose Control".'

It must be hard to find suitable music for a CT scanner.

I was still lying with my arms above my head and the next job was to tattoo marks on my body to ensure that the treatment was always directed at the same place. Also, if I needed more treatment in future, there was a permanent record on my body of the area previously treated, as the body can only stand so much.

I had heard of the 'Blue Tattoo Club' – all of the women who have been marked in this way – so I was disappointed when the radiotherapist arrived with a red tattooing pen. She placed the pen between my breasts as though I was a table. She bent over my body, her nose three inches from my breastbone, her blonde ponytail flopping to the side, and measured me with a ruler, then she took the tattooing pen and marked me permanently between my breasts, once on the right side of my chest and once on the left.

I had mixed feelings about these permanent marks and as I lay there, I could feel my reaction hanging in the balance. Half-naked on a CT scanner is a difficult place to be rational. On one hand, the marks symbolised the passivity of being a cancer patient – I was not asked if I wanted them, I was told I was having them and to lie still while I got them. They also symbolised the permanency of membership of this club. They were a lifelong reminder that the cancer may come back. On the other hand, I remembered the friend in Southern Italy proudly pulling her blouse aside to show me the radiotherapy blue dot on her breast, which she displayed as a badge of survival.

The phrase 'The mark of Cain' flashed through my mind and I tried to remember the story from primary school. Who was Cain and what was his mark? What did it symbolise? Was I being branded with a curse? It was only later that I discovered the mark of Cain was both a curse and a protection from premature death.

I decided to embrace the tattoo marks as another part of my story; my body was already covered in evidence that I have lived a life and these marks were another chapter.

When I broke my arm skiing in my early forties, the bones would not heal and I had pins screwed in for weeks, with an unwieldy external fixator protruding from slits in my forearm. This left three scars, which, ten years later, I had covered with a tattoo of ivy coiling round my wrist and up my arm.

On the back of my leg was a three-inch silver scar from child-hood when I slid my leg into our Austin Princess and a shard of jagged metal sliced through the flesh like a raw pork chop.

There was a wavy scar on my shin from slipping on corrugated iron behind the cow sheds, nearly fifty years ago, trying to keep up with my big cousins.

There was a twenty-year-old scar on my eyebrow from a heavy-handed beautician.

I must still have the episiotomy scar from the birth of my first daughter, although I had never dared to look at it.

And of course, there was the fresh tender scar of the lumpectomy.

Kintsugi is a Japanese method of repairing pottery with a spe-cial lacquer dusted with powdered gold. It translates as 'golden joinery' and leaves seams of gold in the bowl instead of cracks and breaks. The glinting veins tell the story of the pottery, rather than trying to disguise the piece's flaws, and as they gleam and shim-mer they become the best part of the bowl. My scars and tattoo marks were my own *kintsugi*, evidence of my own story.

That night I went to a fiftieth birthday party where an acquaint-ance recoiled when I told him I was being treated for breast cancer. His wife had received the same recall letter from the same mammogram programme to attend the same breast clinic and would find out in two days if she needed a biopsy. 'She'll be fine,' I declared, not having a clue if she would be fine or not, 'she'll be one of the four in five lucky ones.'

I saw the terror on his face; the familiar terror of not knowing if the earth would stay firm beneath your feet.

I realised I was part way along this journey now. I had travelled far enough to be one of the women who looked back and held out a hand, wanting to help those behind, even if my words were false and my smile forced.

My memoir was due for publication in three and a half months and I was keen to narrate the audio book. When I first met my editor, I said the book needed to be narrated in a Lancashire accent. 'In fact, it needs to be me.' And she smiled and agreed.

That had been five months ago, a couple of weeks before my life ricocheted off to Cancerland. Life had had an unreal quality back then – not the unreal quality of cancer but the unreal quality of dreams coming true; having a book deal and going to London to meet your editor and your agent and being invited to your publisher's Summer Party. That kind of unreal quality.

The 2018 heatwave had added to the unreality; the sun shone day after day, warm enough to colour your shoulders, even in Scotland. I was living my dream, not my nightmare.

I had wandered around my publisher's Summer Party at the V&A Museum taking surreptitious selfies, hoping to capture a celebrity writer in the background, tasting my first oyster, sampling the cocktail bar, trying to juggle the canapés and the prosecco and the small talk while not looking giddily, ridiculously delighted. This was the life. I had dreamed of being a writer since I was a child, and in recent years fantasised about saying, 'I'm off to London for lunch with my publisher.' And now the scenario was happening, I was revelling in it.

Then I got cancer.

As I lay on the biopsy bed back in August I had said, 'But I've got a book coming out in February.' And later on that day, when Lizzie the breast care nurse explained that radiotherapy could be completed by Christmas but if chemo were needed it would take another couple of months, I knew in that case we would be cutting it fine. There had been two clear images in my head: one of me at the book launch with hair and one of me at the book launch without hair. Now I knew I would have hair, but I was still nervous that the radiotherapy would make it impossible for me to record the book.

I had been apprehensive about telling work contacts that I had cancer – would they think I would become unreliable? *Would* I become unreliable? Would organisations stop offering me work running writing workshops and doing readings? Would they think I needed to be left alone or that I wouldn't have the time, energy or inclination to work? Being a writer had come so late, it would be cruel for it to vanish again.

But work offers did not dry up; my publisher sent flowers and assured me any remaining editing could be fitted into my schedule – and now they had organised for me to record the audio book in the week between my radiotherapy planning appointment and the radiotherapy sessions beginning.

It was in a small studio a half-hour walk from home in Edinburgh.

I sat in the recording studio alone – me, a glass of water, a microphone, headphones, the manuscript of my book, a reading lamp creating a pool of yellow light around the script. For two full days I read my memoir from start to finish. Every time I stumbled, I paused, went back to the previous full stop and started again. All I could hear was my own voice, loud and clear right behind my eyes, recounting the events that had led to the death by suicide of my little sister; my own voice telling the story of my life and how I had got to here.

Except it was not 'here' any more, because the book had been written before I got cancer.

Occasionally, the sound engineer in his glass bubble asked through the headphones, 'Do you need a break?' But, no, I didn't. It was other-worldly sitting in the darkened studio telling my story to a void, making an account of myself to an echoing space.

And when I got to the end of the book – a hopeful, optimistic ending – I had the urge to lean forward and confide to the micro-phone, 'Yes, but life's an assault course; you survive the scramble through the mud and the struggle with the tangled netting, you inch along the high ropes and think you are on the home straight; then you smack straight into a ten-foot wall.'

Nineteen

When I was told to come off the HRT by breast care nurse Lizzie, I felt bereft, as though my clinging fingers were being prised from the edge of a life raft. I had memories of living with hot flushes and night sweats, which I had initially thought were a debilitating virus, ten years before, and I didn't want them back.

As soon as I stopped taking the HRT, the hot flushes returned, but they were only one or two a day and bearable. I could handle them. I believed it was a case of mind over matter. I remembered a programme about learning to walk on red-hot coals and how the participants had repeated the phrase *Cool Wet Grass* as they placed their feet on embers to convince their brains they were not burning. I consider myself a determined person. If fire walkers could do it, so could I. I would *Cool Wet Grass* my way through the hot flushes.

However, as soon as I started tamoxifen it was a different story. As the drug forced my oestrogen levels to extinction, the hot flushes were fierce and almost constant. Once or twice pre-tamoxifen I recited *Cool Wet Grass* and forced a flush into retreat, but now *Cool Wet Grass* was woefully inadequate.

The term 'hot flush' does not suffice. Until I had my first experience of a hot flush, I thought they were something from a comedy sketch – a Les Dawson punchline. Les Dawson and Roy Barraclough were regulars on television in the seventies, done up in drag, dressed as 'Cissie and Ada', two Lancashire house-wives – grotesque versions of many of the women I met in our Lancashire village shop and local church when I was growing up. They lived in a world of 'roll-ons' and 'gussets', often wearing curlers and pinnies, either with or without dentures. Ada constantly adjusted one bosom, as though it was about to escape, while both 'women' pursed their lips and talked tongue in cheek (literally and figuratively) about sex, death, marriage and everything.

Cissie: On your honeymoon in Blackpool, were you virgo intacta?

Ada: No, we were only B&B.

Folding their arms, tugging their cardigans over their enormous busts, or clutching their handbags, they silently mouthed any words considered too delicate to voice out loud. But that did not include 'hot flushes', which were funny, apparently. In a sketch in which Cissie and Ada were wandering round an art gallery, they stopped to admire a naked Grecian statue.

Ooh, stand back, Cissie, you'll have a flush!

Or when they bent over, showing their bloomers (or as my Grandma called them, 'next week's washing'), they'd straighten up, with, *Ooh, I nearly had a flush.*

To male comedians, the hot flush was a joke at the expense of risible old women.

But these tamoxifen-fuelled monsters were no joke. Repeating *Cool Wet Grass* in the face of one was like fighting a war with a teaspoon.

The flush would begin as a sensation in the sinuses, a pressure in the head, a shifting and prickling around the eyes, a throbbing in the roof of my mouth, all of which quickly became dizzying in intensity. There would be burning along my hairline, a pricking all over my scalp, in front of my ears, round the back of my neck, which seared down my body like a terrible allergic reaction, and yet my skin would not go blotchy, my face would not turn red; sometimes, fine sweat would break out on my forehead, otherwise I appeared normal. But the burning heat crawling over my body was overwhelming and in an enclosed space – a theatre seat or on the bus – the smothering sensation would threaten to trigger a panic attack. There was a terrible urgency to dampen the heat and I would grab anything to fan myself, tearing off clothing and pressing my face against the cold bus windowpanes. I would visualise bare feet on *Cool Wet Grass* and when that failed, conjure images of feet crunching through ice, sinking into five-foot snow drifts, then whole naked bodies plunging into Arctic ice holes – all to no avail, as the heat intensified, burning me up and suffusing me with nausea. And this sensation, this apparently 'comic' hot flush with the prickling burning of an allergic reaction, the overwhelming anxiety of a panic attack and the sweaty nausea of a hangover, would engulf me several times an hour, all day and all night.

The nights were the worst. I would rest on a cool pillow and drop off only to be woken minutes later, hot from head to foot, kicking off covers, peeling off pyjamas, desperate to save myself from being burnt alive. It was a medieval hell: tortured on a bed of glowing coals, prodded awake by devils with forks.

I would stumble to the bathroom, pressing my face and arms against the wall to leach the cool from it. Standing barefoot on cold tiles, in this unheated bathroom in Scotland, in winter, I would visualise the infusion of coldness up my legs and the draining away of the heat into the floor.

I would perch on the side of the freezing metal bath as moonlight shone through the shutter slats, creating a pattern like the bars of a prison.

I was trapped, unable to escape from myself, even to sleep. Unaccustomed to a body that was apparently mine; a body possessed by the goddess of fire.

I was untethered from everything familiar.

Living with these loud, clamouring and constant tamoxifen side effects was intensely claustrophobic. I had lost my ability to be quiet and retreat into my own head. My head and body now had squatters that were spending twenty-four hours a day smashing the place up while the small part of the original me hid in the garden and peered terrified from behind the dustbin.

I would return from the bathroom and lie on top of the duvet fanning myself, counting through the hot flush like I had counted through the contractions when I was in labour with my daughters. With a contraction, I knew when I got to around forty it would begin to abate, the pain would ebb and I would come back to this world, but these engulfing hot flushes went on and on. It was difficult to get to the end of counting because the counting never ended.

Three, four, five minutes and I would still be burning and counting, and then, just as suddenly, would come the chills. A mad scramble for the covers, trying to shield every inch of skin from the night air as the shivering started and the cold crawled up and down my back, arms and legs, no matter how many blankets I piled on.

My mother used to describe a shudder as 'someone walking over my grave', but this all-over body shiver was much more than that, it was someone dragging rusty metal over my grave.

I mentioned the hot flushes to the oncologist, and she looked at me with sympathy: 'Coming off HRT to go on tamoxifen can be rocky. Stick with it.'

She suggested drinking cold water in the evening rather than hot drinks – another small pleasure ruled out along with hot baths, warm blankets, polo neck jumpers, cosy scarves, zipped-up fleeces, wine, spicy food, tucking the duvet under my chin, even having the cat on my lap – all gone.

I searched online for advice about hot flushes: *Go to sleep in a damp shirt* (a 'cure' surely as bad as the illness), *don't fan or take off layers – it makes it worse*, advice that reminded me of a teenage boyfriend who bought me my first vindaloo and insisted I drank nothing with it. 'Water makes it hotter,' he said, laughing as my eyes streamed.

The most consistent advice: *take HRT*.

'I hate being cold,' said a friend with a particular knack of always saying the wrong thing, 'I'm looking forward to hot flushes.'

Twenty

Arriving for my first radiotherapy session, I looked up at the Cancer Centre sign and saw it was not gold at all, but grimy white and certainly not something that would look at home in a disco. Was it the winter sun that had made it glow? I was disconcerted; it was as though the world was telling me not to trust my own senses.

In the radiotherapy waiting room, there was a semi-circle of chairs around two coffee tables, one of which carried a *Scotsman* newspaper with the headline: 'Cancer deaths rise in Scotland as mortality rates down 10 per cent over decade'. The universe was apparently organising a running commentary on my life to heighten the unreality. I ignored the newspaper – it would seem rude to read such a story in front of all these people with cancer.

Later I Googled it and discovered that 'Cancer charities are demanding the number of staff in the NHS is increased "urgently" after new figures showed a rise in deaths last year'. There were apparently 16,105 deaths caused by cancer in Scotland in 2017, up from 15,813 the previous year. But even though the total number of deaths was up, the overall mortality rates were down in the past decade, from 358 deaths per 100,000 people in 2007 to 321 deaths per 100,000 in 2017. I found it hard to get my mind around the statistics, but I think it meant the news was both good and bad.

The newspaper yelled its mixed messages to the room, un-picked up, as though none of us had seen it. Instead, I got out my notebook to write down the defining characteristics of a radiotherapy waiting room. I would be spending a long time in here so I might as well not waste it.

The lady beside me was knitting a jumper in all colours of the rainbow on tiny needles, her wool tucked into a shopping bag at her feet. In my notebook I wrote 'Madame Defarge', the name of the character from Dickens' *A Tale of Two Cities* who sat by the guillotine encoding the names of those who must die into her knitting.

That was the trouble with having cancer; it made everything into a drama. Nothing was normal any more. Nothing was everyday. Everything was heightened. Everything was *more*. Everything was swept up into my cancer story as I searched the mundane for meaning. A grubby white sign became disco-gold, a knitting lady in a waiting room became Madame Defarge chronicling the doomed.

I was about to write, 'They were the best of times they were the worst of times', when the knitting lady's nose gushed with blood and I scrambled for tissues as she sat, head back and mouth agape, not unlike a salmon on a fishmonger's slab, or indeed a severed head in a basket.

I hoped she had not glimpsed what I had written.

She was soon mopped up and I angled my notebook away from her and continued to jot down details. The man opposite was reading *End Game*, by David Baldacci. Another man was hidden behind the *Daily Record*, with the front-page headline 'Please end my Hallowe'en nightmare', and back-page headline 'Shape up or I'm out'. One or two of the patients chatted among themselves, obviously having met here before. Some fiddled with their phones, or iPads, or stared into space in silence, biting their nails. A man arrived in a wheelchair with a drip attached, pushed by an orderly.

A little further up the corridor, I glimpsed a thin, ill-looking man, head down, sitting alone. He looked up and I averted my eyes, then glanced back. Who was he? What was his story? I began to create a poignant narrative for him – he was so thin ... so alone – only to spot his badge and realise he was a volunteer running one of the snack bars.

I was surrounded by posters: *Please work with us not against us.* Did cancer patients abuse the staff who were helping them? Several times over the weeks I meant to ask one of the radiotherapists, but there was never time.

On the water filter in red capital letters: *PLEASE DISPOSE OF YOUR EMPTY CUPS IN THE BINS PROVIDED.* Another poster: *Are you taking strong painkillers for cancer pain? Are you also taking Paracetamol?* A fluttering handwritten notice: *Please ensure that patients have priority over seating in this waiting area.*

This was a quiet room with LOUD walls.

Most of the patients were elderly, one or two were in their fifties and occasionally there was someone younger.

When the knitting lady was called for her appointment she trilled, 'One more stitch to the end of the row', before bundling her knitting into her bag and hurrying off.

I was in the waiting room for 'LA4', but it took me another three weeks to ask what 'LA' stood for. It was a linear accelerator, the machine used for external beam radiation cancer treatment and which would deliver high-energy X-rays to the region of my tumour.

As it was my first time, I had a meeting with a young male radiotherapist, who gave me a bag of creams and told me how to care for my skin to try to prevent skin damage. He reassured me the radiation could not move around my body or be transferred to anyone else. 'So, don't worry about that,' he said, and I realised it was the only thing I hadn't been worrying about.

He gave me strict instructions on how to lie on the treatment bed: I must not try to help the radiographers by adjusting my position. The adjustments needed were minute and I would only overcompensate and make it worse. It was my job to lie dead still and be adjusted.

Like the room with the CT scanner, the radiotherapy room was as cold as a chiller cabinet. Being chilled to the bone would become a defining characteristic of the whole radiotherapy experience.

Again, I went behind a small semi-circular curtain and removed my upper clothing and, clutching the cover cloth, I emerged and clambered onto the treatment bed. Today the music was disco – Chaka Khan singing 'I'm Every Woman'.

'We had an iPod but it broke,' said one of the radiotherapists. 'We find the disco CD is a big hit.'

I lay with my arms above my head in the stirrups. There was no blue-sky screen on the ceiling here to help me escape.

An arm of the machine lowered itself to within a foot of my body and shone red laser beams across my breasts. This strangely sentient machine had me in its cross hairs. The young male radiographer tugged at my torso this way and that to line me up, using the tattoo marks. I remembered my instructions not to help – which was hard when you have been raised never to be a nuisance. I lay as still as a body on a slab. The radiographer's hands were freezing, and I tried not to shiver. I told him how cold they were, and he laughed. 'Yes,' he said.

Once in position, I shallow breathed to minimise movement. The radiographers said they would go into the control room while the machine delivered the radiotherapy and would return in a few minutes. An alarm went off and they jogged from the room.

Hearing the honking alarm and their receding footsteps was the loneliest feeling.

In the freezing room, the machine began to whir and click and move. I could not turn my head but sensed another arm of the machine coming up on my left. It was like the mating dance of a giant robot; what writer Jenni Diski, when she was being treated for cancer, described as a *danse macabre*. Whir. Click. Move. I was still barely breathing, trying not to shiver or twitch. I concentrated on working out which disco track was playing but the sound was turned down too low.

Afterwards I dressed quickly, aware of the queue of people outside waiting for their chance to dance with the robot. I asked if I could take a photograph of the two young women radiotherapists there when I emerged from behind the curtain, and they posed, smiling sweetly, alongside the machine. Taking a photograph was apparently not unusual: 'Some people like to document their journeys,' said one.

Studying the picture of their kind faces later, I looked forward to getting to know them. My friend said her elderly mother enjoyed her days out to the radiotherapy unit and made lots of friends, but as the days ticked by, I rarely saw the same person twice and I never did get to know them.

Sometimes the wait was longer if the machine broke down, which it seemed to do quite often because if the safety features were triggered, they required a lengthy resetting. Then, I would be transferred to another machine with different staff altogether.

But every room was as cold as the last. 'The machines like it,' explained one radiographer, but another said, 'Yeah, they can never get the air con right in here.' My friend who had treatment during a heatwave told me, 'Ooh, I was boiling in there.'

Cello drove me to hospital every day, despite me insisting I was fine to go alone. In fact, I was filled with such fear that I was not fine to go alone.

The drive out West became routine, through the Georgian tenements, the town houses, the posh Georgian villas, past the Royal Botanic Garden and the grandiose Fettes College to the architectural wasteland of the hospital.

As each day passed, more Christmas decorations appeared in shops and Christmas tree lights flashed in tenement windows. One day a Christmas appeal by a cancer charity came on the car radio. *Help us support people with cancer to live life as fully as they can...*

'But that's not for me, is it?' I asked, 'that's not about people like me?'

Cello shook his head, 'No,' he answered, 'not like you', although at that moment I don't think either of us had a clue what I was on about. I think being someone who had lost the privilege of good health was too frightening to accept. From well to sick, from having a private body to a public one, from person to patient, from observer to observed, from doer to done-to, from giver to taker, it changed who I thought I was.

We cut it finer every day until I was dashing straight from the car into the Cancer Centre as Cello queued for the car park. I shot through the hospital, slowing down to scan the organic vegetable stall, glancing at the free second-hand books, and heading down the sloping corridor to LA4.

As routine as it became, though, I never forgot, not for a second, that I was in the Cancer Centre. Even on the loo I was faced with the notice: *Advice for Patients: Using the toilet while on chemotherapy,* which cautioned that chemo drugs could be passed in bodily fluids and may harm other patients.

I became used to the routine of waiting my turn, my name being called, stripping off behind the flimsy curtain, clutching the cover cloth as I clambered onto the bed, giving my name and date of birth then lying down with my arms in the stirrups like an inanimate object. But unfortunately, from that point the proceedings ceased to be routine and became a daily agony because I have hypermobile joints that reacted terribly to the position I had to maintain.

My hypermobile joints had in the past been something to show off about: they are loose joints that extend easily and painlessly beyond the normal range due to weak ligaments.

As a child I was able to do the lotus position with ease, which impressed my mother – not a woman easily impressed – who herself attempted throughout the 1970s, with a series of yoga night classes and *Yoga for All* books, to do the lotus position and failed. Night after night on the hearth rug in front of the open fire as *Look North* blared in the background, she tried to get her right foot onto her left thigh and then to lower her right knee, and always failed – as I watched, sitting in the full lotus with my arms in prayer position behind my back, then as she gritted her teeth I'd ceremoniously lower my forehead to the ground. To her credit, she never told me to clear off. Back then I could get my leg behind my head and touch my thumb flat to my wrist. I was proud of my bendy joints.

Having hypermobile joints was why I had laughed at the radiographer's question at the measuring-up session as to whether I could get my arms above my head. Me? Stalwart of the over-fifties yoga class, have trouble getting my arms above my head? I should think not. Surely my bendy joints would make the positioning on the radiotherapy bed easy.

It was not to be.

The agony started three days in – a piercing pain deep inside the shoulder joint that persisted throughout the day and night. I asked one of the radiographers about seeing a physio. 'Oh, yes, the department used to have one – but we don't any more.'

She suggested I took painkillers before I arrived for the daily session, so I dug out the tramadol my mother had refused to take when she was dying of cancer – now ten years old and six years out of date – and I took that. It did not help. I lay on the bed still in agony and now tramadol-dizzy.

As well as the pain, there was the terrible sensation that my right shoulder was about to pop out of joint as I lay there in the freezing cold, trying not to cry, trying not to shiver, as the staff ran out of the room and the machine began its weird clicking dance.

The radiotherapists would work as quickly as they could, putting the B&Q metal ruler and red felt pens between my breasts as they nudged me into position, then marking me up in line with the laser beams. Once I was in position, they rested the crepe paper 'cover cloth' on my chest like my mother covering a cake with a tea towel to keep the flies off. But the ten minutes with my arms up in the stirrups and my right shoulder screaming in agony felt like hours.

On music-less days, when the disco CD was silent, I stared at the ceiling memorising what I could see to take my mind off the searing pain. I gazed in misery at the ceiling tiles that looked like the old flammable ones that used to peel off our bathroom ceiling in the farmhouse and two air-conditioning vents that intermittently blew cold air on me, making the 'cover cloth' ripple on my chest and me shiver even more. All the while, the eye of the machine, a two-foot circle, winked and blinked and whirred and clicked. It took immense self-control not to panic as the days progressed and the pain worsened.

Cello got me an appointment with a sports physio and when he said, 'Hello, Catherine, how are you?' in a kind voice, I burst into tears and couldn't speak.

He told me I had damaged my rotator cuff and had knock-on damage to a nerve running down my arm, which wouldn't get better until the radiotherapy was finished. He told me his wife had been treated for breast cancer several years ago. As I lay face down on the treatment table, with my right breast throbbing from the surgery, I told him I was lucky/unlucky; lucky the cancer was caught early, unlucky to get it at all, and he replied, 'No, you were just unlucky.'

His response was a relief. I agreed; it was terrible luck.

I was tired of being positive.

Twenty

After three visits to the physio, I resented cancer for costing me money as well as time, pain, anguish and terror. Then I stumbled on an article from the United States with a section on 'Understanding the Costs Associated with Cancer' and its link, 'Help for People without Health Insurance', and it hit me how very much worse everything could be. With its talk of 'patient financial counsellors' and 'health insurance marketplace', and its advice to 'see if your hospital or cancer centre has any kind of discount program for people without health insurance', it was a horror story, and I acknowledged again how lucky/unlucky I was.

In a review meeting with a senior radiotherapist, a fortnight into the treatment, I asked about the exact area being treated, so I would know which area to keep out of direct sunlight in future. The radiotherapist rooted in my file then slapped an A4 sheet of paper onto the desk. Cello and I stared at it. It was an image of a topless woman, from the chin to the waist. 'Is that me?' I asked, utterly taken aback. I had no idea there were 'photographs' of me on the machine. It was ghostly and grey; it had the air of an image taken surreptitiously with night-vision goggles, possibly through the sights of a gun; and there was something dusty and 'of the grave' about it. Something 'true crime' about it: the arms above the head, lying naked, like a victim, trussed up. Something pornographic about it too.

I stared at it, speechless. The radiotherapist did not see my shock and continued, 'It's the area from the clavicle down between the breasts across the bottom of your breast and up your right side to the middle of your armpit.'

She said it should always be covered in factor 50 or, even better, a high-necked T-shirt. So much for the new bikinis. I continued to gawp at the image and Cello leaned over the desk again: 'You look good though,' he said. I was lost for words, so the meeting ended, and it was only later that I wished I had taken a photograph of it to take the image back into my possession, to reclaim a part of me, a naked, vulnerable part, too intimate to be left lying in a hospital filing cabinet.

That night, as Cello and I watched a police drama, I realised that a cancer diagnosis was like being thrust into the criminal justice system: a huge, dehumanising bureaucracy, with no choices, little dignity or privacy, all control removed, overwhelming and terrifying. Like the prisoner on the television who was currently having his mug shots taken, I too longed for it all to be a mistake and to hear the door creaking open to let me out into the fresh air.

Cello and I were side by side, but we were living in different worlds because we were living in different bodies.

Twenty-One

Part way through radiotherapy, I went on a writing weekend. The hot flushes were fierce, the pain in my shoulder took my breath away, headaches crawled round my temples and up my sinuses and I got random waves of nausea, like gut-punches, that left me gagging.

I did not join in the prosecco and gin drinking with the other writers because I knew it would make me feel worse. I barely slept. I lay awake hour after hour in an unfamiliar bed with dark thoughts swirling. A deep depression and hopelessness descended. As I stared blindly into the blackness, my thoughts became crystal clear: there was no point in anything because everything could be snatched away in a second. The pointlessness of making plans, of having dreams, of working towards anything was overwhelming. The voices in my head were clear: it was all for nothing.

Throughout the night the hot flushes were replaced with cold chills that travelled up and down my body like the frozen fingers of a concert pianist.

The next day we did a writing workshop on the theme of 'lost' and I jotted down: 'Three towns, two careers, one farm, six cars, five cats, four cousins, one sister, one mother, and now myself. All gone.'

I told some of the other women about the unbearable side effects of the tamoxifen. I explained it worked by reducing the action of oestrogen in the body. One of them said, 'Oh, you'll get hairs on your chin next. Then a dry vagina; I have a poem about dry vaginas.' She rooted in her bag and brought out her notebook. 'Shall I read it?'

When I mentioned this poem to friends, I was surprised by how many women, both younger and older, said, 'Oh yes, that's a thing.' Another issue so taboo I had not realised it *was* an issue.

When I returned from the writing weekend, I was exhausted and distraught. At home I had yet another sleepless night lying in the pitch black under the sloping bedroom ceiling. Lara, who loves the small hours, says, 'There are no rules at 4am like there are at 4pm', and I wished I could find the upside of being awake at this, the darkest hour. I heard seagulls on the roof, the night bus, the crash of illegal late-night glass recycling from the restaurant opposite. I heard my husband breathing deeply, asleep within seconds of lying down, and I heard an inner voice say: *You didn't expect life to be like this, did you?*

I had recently stumbled on a study suggesting that breast cancer may be more likely to recur in women who suffer from insomnia.

I lay awake all night worrying about lying awake all night worrying.

I recalled being in labour with Lara – another long night lying awake in the dark beside a sleeping husband. My waters broke on a Saturday morning and twice that day we were sent home from the hospital because they said labour was not far enough advanced. I knew the contractions were as powerful as when I had given birth to Nina, but the midwives told me my labour was not established and I was better off at home for the time being. As I left the hospital in agony for the second time, I felt I was being gaslit by the medical profession.

What the midwives did not realise was that Lara was a 'stargazer baby', lying back-to-back with me rather than facing down, as is the norm. This meant the contractions were strong, painful and regular, but my cervix was dilating only slowly, a never-ending agony for little result. At the time, Nina was almost three and obsessed with Disney's *Snow White* – so I lay in bed at home all Saturday night with *Hi-ho, Hi-ho. It's off to work we go…* ringing round and round in my head. I counted contractions throughout the pitch-black small hours, the number of the seconds flickering like neon in my head. *Hi-HO!*

When Lara was eventually born in hospital the following evening, the newly qualified midwife who delivered her gave a shriek as she emerged face up rather than face down. 'I should have known which way she was lying!' she said. She apologised that I had torn. 'I should have stopped it!' Despite needing an hour's stitching up, I felt nothing but goodwill towards this woman with the tired dark circles around her eyes, who may have got it wrong but had been gentle and kind throughout.

Now, twenty years later, here was another endless, sleepless night. Eventually I gave up trying to sleep and lay with the light from my phone making my eyes water as I Googled and browsed, over and over, endless scrolling.

Tamoxifen + hot flushes
Tamoxifen + nausea
Tamoxifen + joint pain
Tamoxifen + weight gain
Tamoxifen + headaches
Tamoxifen + fatigue
Tamoxifen + hair loss
Tamoxifen + mood swings
Tamoxifen + dry skin
Tamoxifen + memory loss
Tamoxifen + confusion
Tamoxifen + depression
Tamoxifen + stroke
Tamoxifen + liver damage
Tamoxifen + blood clots

I tumbled head over heels down an internet rabbit hole ricocheting from reputable sites run by the NHS and respected charities to all kinds of so-called 'experts', but I could find no good news about life on tamoxifen. I pored over forums and blogs:

...my body hurts, I can't sleep. I am angry all the time...

...I have hot flushes, thinning hair, overwhelming fatigue, confusion, strange thinking...

...I feel horrible ... my brain hurts ... I have trouble thinking.

Someone mentioned their 'Tamoxi-belly' and others described weight gain they blamed on tamoxifen. This struck fear – an actual physical pain – into me and I lay in the dark crying, suffused by panic and shame.

Tamoxifen + weight gain
Tamoxifen + weight gain
Tamoxifen + weight gain

Twenty-Two

As a child I was skinny. My legs were thin with knobbly knees, 'like a calf' according to my big sister. An aunt called me 'Twiggy', which I knew was a compliment. Twiggy, snappy, sticky, Twiggy. 'I wish I was...' added my aunt, heartfelt.

I was glad not to be a 'fatty' because nobody wanted to be a 'Ten-Ton Tessie'. Fat was comical and embarrassing. You only had to compare the reactions to Hattie Jacques and Barbara Windsor in the *Carry On* films to know that. Slimness brought approval; fatness brought ridicule. Fat was isolating, different and shaming. Fat was *wrong*.

These were the messages from society, and I was receptive to them.

Until puberty I was skin and bone, shot through with that feeling of freedom, of lightness, of flying. I was flexible and nimble and could run, jump, swing, climb and balance with ease. Farm kids were the original parkour kids, but instead of buildings, we negotiated bales, fences, gates, hedges, trees, woods, ditches and barns, chasing over and under, around and across.

Farm kids are more suited to being outside than in. When I holidayed in a retired aunt's bungalow, my uncle told me off for throwing myself at the sofa rather than sitting down 'like a lady', and threatened to put me over his knee if I ended up pulling a button off the new leather-look sofa. By the end of the week I had been trained to perch on the sofa edge, dress smoothed to my knees like the Queen herself.

It was a relief to get back to the freedom of the farm, where I loved to move – or at least, I did until puberty.

Then that sense of freedom vanished and was replaced with self-consciousness and the beginning of a lifetime of wanting to be smaller, firmer, less jiggly, less embarrassing, less shameful, less obvious – just less – to be neater, tidier, more controlled.

I began to clamp my arms against my chest to stop it being painful and embarrassing when I ran – it no longer looked more fun to be a girl than a boy.

Also gone was the prepubescent untroubled, guilt-free eating. I remembered watching the crumbs from my mother's Energen roll – a ball of baked cellulose marketed as a diet aid and tasting like crunchy fresh air – falling like dust onto her plate, as everyone else tucked into a delicious hearty meal prepared by her. My mother spent her life thinking about 'slimming' and wanting to lose two stones and now here I was, a teenager always wanting to lose five pounds. I would ask, 'Is this fattening?', to which she would reply ominously, '*All* food is fattening.'

There was only one kind of acceptable woman and that was a thin one. Apparently, thin equalled happy and successful. If only I could lose a few pounds I would be … happier how? If thinness was the answer, what was the question? Except I *didn't* question it. There was a sense that women must take control of their body shape, which could never be left to nature or to chance. We were responsible for being attractive and acceptable. It was normal for women to be dissatisfied with their body shape and to be dieting, planning a diet or bemoaning a failed diet. I remember hearing one woman say, 'It's the hunger I can't stand', and not finding this deprivation wrong or strange in any way. Bodies were things to be fixed, and the act of fixing was a constant struggle.

'Fat is a state of mind,' said Susie Orbach in *Fat is a Feminist Issue*, a book published in 1976 but unfortunately not read by me for another generation. So, in 1983, aged twenty, weighing just over nine and a half stones, at five foot seven and wearing size ten jeans, I joined my first slimming club.

Twenty-Two

I queued up, shoes off, in a down-at-heel community centre to be weighed in. Seeing the needle fall below ten stones, the hard-faced woman with a smoker's cough who ran the class barked, 'You've only just arrived in time, haven't you?' I laughed, shame-faced – that hovering ten stone was indeed horrifying.

I was put on something called *The Human Diet, for those with up to a stone to lose.* The diet sheet, confidently subtitled *Where your weight problems end,* was a joyless document with a section of 'Light Meals' that included 'Liver with Onion and Gravy' – but, where the recipe should have been, it said: '1 packet Birds Eye Liver with Onion and Gravy.' Another suggestion was 'Soup: 1 sachet Batchelors Cup-a-Soup Special with Croutons.' For 'Main Meals' it included 'Prawn Curry: 1 portion Vesta Prawn Curry' or 'Shepherd's Pie: 8oz Findus Shepherd's Pie'.

This starvation 1,000-calorie a day diet may have been about thinness, but it was nothing to do with health or happiness and was a far cry from the home-made, home-grown food I had been brought up on.

The ethos of the group seemed to be one of bullying and humiliation to 'encourage and inspire' weight loss – not unlike the parody slimming group 'Fat Fighters' in the television series *Little Britain* years later. It was not approved of for you to leave after weigh-in – they preferred you to stay and join in the conversation about food: what new 'slimming' food was on the market, what snacks you could get away with while watching television, which foods could be frozen (bananas, chocolates, grapes) to make them harder to eat. For people trying to eat less, they spent a long time focusing on food.

If there was a week when I put on weight, the barking woman stuck a sticker of a pink pig in my weighing-in book. Even Fat Fighters didn't do that. Did the barking woman have a cigarette dangling from the corner of her mouth, or have I imagined that?

When I told my boyfriend about the pink pigs, he laughed so hard I thought he might crash the car.

Without realising it, I had become immersed in 'diet culture' – a phrase I did not hear for many more years. I assumed the slimming industry was benevolent, there to help me overcome a personal failing and provide rules to help me muster the will-power to go hungry to achieve slimness.

After abandoning that first slimming group, life continued with diet recipe books, diet magazines full of 'before and after' photographs for 'inspiration', food that was low-calorie, lo-cal, lite, lean, fat-free, guilt-free, steamed vegetables, vegetable soup, vegetables with boil-in-the-bag fish, vegetables cooked in a 'fat-less frying pan', lunch of cottage cheese (what Susie Orbach calls the *slimmer's methadone*) eaten at my office desk, nights in the pub staring at a slimline orange.

The preoccupation with food intake took much energy and time: what had I eaten? What would I eat next? What should I have eaten? What shouldn't I have eaten? How would I last until tomorrow without eating again? Like the slimmers at the club, for someone trying to cut down on food, I spent an inordinate amount of time thinking about it.

I avoided anything 'sinfully delicious', 'indulgent' or 'luxury' until such time as I thought I deserved a 'treat' or had something to celebrate – then I ate Chinese takeaway, or home-made curry or Kentucky Fried Chicken until I could barely move, or if alcohol was more important, I'd go to the corner shop for a bottle of cider and a Mars Bar, occasionally getting dressed at midnight and going in search of an all-night garage to buy chocolate … then, after eating it, I would plan the next diet. There was always a hefty price to pay for enjoying food. I was convinced the only alternative to these strictures was chaos.

All the time, my jeans were never bigger than a size ten, but the fear of getting fat was real. I lived alone and often kept no food in the house at all. In a fatphobic world, I stuck pictures of fat women on my fridge to frighten me and pictures of thin women to inspire me. When I went to stay with a friend, I took my own Ryvita. My friend Carole still remembers coming for tea and being given lettuce butties.

A friend's mother said, 'When I was a teenager there was none of this calorie counting, we just went and played tennis', and I thought, she doesn't *understand*.

I developed an in-built calorie counter, always on duty, and knew the calorific values of everything from a polo mint (six calories) upwards. Lightning-fast calculations of calories was my superpower. I weighed myself every morning and the difference of a pound more or a pound less set the tone for the day – a tone of success or failure. When the fizzy pop 'One Cal' was launched in the mid-eighties, I welcomed it like an artificial-tasting manna from heaven. Surely there would soon be calorie-free food?

I kept food diaries; many days abandoned by mid-afternoon when I had already exceeded 1,000 calories. Also scattered around the house were endless listings of daily weigh-ins, one listing containing two weigh-ins per day – one for each set of scales in the house.

Although I feared getting fat and longed to be less, I *loved* food. I loved the taste of food and the sensation of being full. I loved the social aspect of food, of family meals and eating out to celebrate. It was all or nothing, bingeing or dieting, hungry or stuffed, an intense compulsive involvement with food.

When I met up with friends, a normal greeting was, 'You look great, have you lost weight?' It was considered polite to ask.

These were the early days of Princess Diana as a public figure. She was two years older than me and I watched agog as the world obsessed about her weight, her fashion sense, her hair, her demeanour, her body language, but mostly her weight. It was probably a good thing that in the eighties I didn't know about bulimia (gorging and vomiting) and learned about it only when Princess Diana talked of it a decade later.

Unknowingly, I had already encountered it: in my first week at university, aged twenty-five, I met a frail girl who told me she always ate an apple before every meal so she could eat whatever else she wanted, then vomit it all back up, stopping only when the regurgitated apple reappeared and she was sure her stomach was empty. I was baffled and uncomprehending – how could eating be such torture? The girl disappeared from university the week after never to be seen again.

I never considered myself to have disordered eating because I never took slimming pills, I never vomited or purged, I never relied on crash diets or meal replacements. I never cut out whole food groups. I ate so many salads and vegetables I considered my diet healthy and this vigilance and phobia about fat to be a normal part of every woman's life. Surely everyone did this?

As the years passed, the media continued its obsession with Princess Diana's body, and I read every article. I remember the glee from the press when the paparazzi snapped 'cellulite' on her thighs. 'Princess Perfect's battle with cellulite,' said one; 'Princess Lumpy Legs,' said another. Eventually a 'deeply hurt' Diana felt compelled to refute this and say the 'cellulite' was the imprint of a wicker bar stool.

Cellulite is part of the female body; it has always been there – Rubens painted it five hundred years ago – but in the late twentieth century it became another nuance in the shaming of women and their lumpy, bumpy, dimpled flesh. Newspapers and women's magazines had a field day: 'helpful' treatments and remedies were offered – useless and expensive creams, massages, diets – including the advice 'never eat a sausage, cheese and biscuits or cake'. Cellulite was graded from 'orange peel' to 'cottage cheese' to 'mattress', so you could appreciate the size and scope of your 'problem'.

The media hounded and judged Diana constantly with this sort of madness, and by extension they hounded and judged every other young woman in the country.

Gaining weight during pregnancy had not worried me because a pregnancy bump is rock hard, not soft fat – but that changes once the baby is born. One of the disappointments of not being able to breastfeed my first daughter was the (false) promise that breastfeeding would reduce my post-birth weight. After breastfeeding my second baby for six months and still weighing the same as the day I gave birth, I went to Weightwatchers and dieted back to just over nine stone – the weight I'd been on my wedding day.

As a new mother, I was regularly made aware of my babies' weights by the health visitor, who seemed to care about little else. Both babies had luscious rolls of fat on their thighs but apparently this put them in the 'higher percentiles'. I was given a book so I could plot on a graph exactly how fat my babies were. I felt a twisting panic as their weights bumped along the outer limits of 'acceptable'.

As they grew, they were not fat, but I worried in case they became fat and were bullied.

I also worried in case they realised I was worried.

At primary school they told me of children being humiliated about their weight, including by the PE teacher, who remarked to the fat, unsporty boy who was a carer for his disabled mother, 'Stop talking! You're like a parrot! Except I wouldn't want *you* sitting on my shoulder.'

I bought a book called *Fit Kids* that contained a photograph of a fat child in trunks playing in the sea with the words 'Sometimes I feel left out' photoshopped over him. Around the edge of the photograph are calculations of my daughters' BMI scores – '21.6', '18.12', '21.9' anxiously scribbled by me over the years.

As my mother had passed on her body insecurity to me, looking back I was afraid I had done the same to my daughters. Asking her now, Nina reassures me it was not as bad as I feared, telling me, 'I didn't know "slim" could be a verb until I saw some old *Jackie* magazines from the seventies.'

Then came the early menopause and I put on a stone in weeks before I understood what was happening, watching helplessly as my weight rose day by day. It was frightening that this fundamental part of me was suddenly beyond my control.

As my weight went up, it was the first thing I thought about in the morning, while the last thing I thought about at night was all the food I regretted eating, and how I would do better tomorrow. I was uncomfortable in all of my clothes. I went to a party and kept my coat on all night. Lara told me I needed to stop wearing baggy clothes and get something more fitted because I looked like a 'big bag of Mum'. I began to resent nights out involving eating, feeling trapped in them.

I went to the GP about my weight gain before the early menopause had been diagnosed. He was a locum doctor, a huge man wedged into a swivel chair. 'You can't expect to be the same weight as you used to be,' he said, and I left, dismissed and told off, but thinking, 'I'm forty-two, why not?'

After several years of feeling as though I was walking around in a fat suit, I joined another slimming group. I went to the weekly weigh-in in my lightest clothes, starving and dehydrating myself all day until I had been on the scales. I once saw another slimmer removing her stud earrings before climbing onto the scales, and I laughed to myself, until I remembered I had considered coming with no knickers on.

Slowly over a year I lost a stone and a half. I reached this target the week I was diagnosed with cancer. But the Frankie Boyle joke 'You're so unlucky I bet you reach your target weight at Weightwatchers the week you are diagnosed with cancer' doesn't work in the way I suspect Frankie intended it to. People assume cancer means thinness, cancer means wasting away and gauntness, they think it means weight loss whether you like it or not, but in fact many women diagnosed with breast cancer gain weight, especially those on hormone treatment like me.

Tamoxifen + weight gain

Reading about this probable weight gain during my frantic midnight Google searches felt like another punishment.

I mentioned this fear of weight gain to a friend who told me off – saying I was being cruel to burden myself with this worry instead of being grateful to my body for its service over the years. I knew I sounded ridiculous to her, trivial and ungrateful, but I could not help it. I knew treating the cancer was what mattered rather than putting on a few pounds, but losing that stone and a half had made me feel like me again. That stone and a half made the difference between living in the right body and living in the wrong body.

I was used to weighing myself every day, but now it became every morning and every night; then each time I got up in the night – squinting at the scales in the moonlight, trying to stop the creak as I stepped on it from waking anyone up – seeing what difference having a pee made. I no longer used scales with a needle – they were not accurate enough. I had to know my weight to a tenth of a pound. I would get off and on again to see if it made the reading go down. I would delay getting dressed in the morning to see if another hour made any difference.

I stuck to the slimming club regime and when, despite that, my weight crept up a few pounds after starting the tamoxifen, I binned the bags of Revels and went to the Vue chocolate-less.

I was terrified of cancer, and of it coming back, but only a small step behind that was the terror of getting fat.

Twenty-Three

By my late teens I had gained a veneer of body confidence by realising I was attractive to men. To be noticed could be a good thing or a bad thing, but it became what I expected.

I overcompensated for the round shoulders I had developed as a self-conscious thirteen-year-old by forcing my shoulders up and back, thinking I was standing correctly. In fact, I was holding them rigid, making the muscles in my shoulders so sore they hurt to the touch. For years I thought everyone had shoulders that made them cry.

Looks were everything; I ran for buses and went shopping in four-inch heels, taking it for granted that my feet would be agonising by evening. The muscles in my calves began to shorten and my Achilles tendons stiffened until walking barefoot was painful. It was worth it. Going out in flat shoes was unthinkable. They were not fashionable, but more importantly they were not sexy.

I wore slim-fitting pencil skirts for work, constantly holding my stomach muscles tight and flat, making my breathing shallow because god forbid that my stomach should be rounded.

I was physically uncomfortable in my body and clothes but accepted that that was the price you paid for sex appeal.

Depending on who it came from, I found certain male attention validating – without realising it was self-esteem built on sand. It never occurred to me to question why I needed that validation at all.

When I was eighteen, I got a job as a barmaid in a traditional copper-topped tables, ornamental tankards kind of pub. I was a good-looking, big-breasted, dark-haired teenager. Every time I sold a packet of peanuts to one of the middle-aged men who lined the bar, the removal of the bag revealed a little more of the picture beneath – a good-looking, big-breasted, dark-haired teenager in a bikini.

If no one wanted serving I stood at the side of the bar reading a book, trying to keep it out of sight. No, said the landlord, go and chat with the men. That's what they are here for. That's what *you* are here for: to look nice, to smile and to listen.

I wasn't even offended, only disappointed that I couldn't read my book. Books were more interesting than half-drunk middle-aged men – even the copy of *Valley of the Dolls* I found at a jumble sale, in which a young woman with breast cancer put her full make-up on, arranged herself prettily on the bed and killed herself so she wouldn't have to continue living with an imperfect body. But I wasn't surprised I was expected to be decorative and pleasing to men behind the bar because that was what the world was apparently about.

Of course, it was impossible to control who responded to the sex appeal I valued so highly, or how. Sometimes the attention came from the right men in the right way, and I enjoyed it.

Flicking through my 1983 diary, from when I was nineteen, I found: 'A man in the market smiled and told his friend I was beautiful. I walked home smiling.'

That was the kind of male attention that boosted my confidence because it 'proved' my attractiveness and desirability. The fact I was entitled to walk around town without unsolicited comments from strange men never occurred to me. Why I needed to have my attractiveness validated by a man I never pondered, nor the man's apparent divine right to judge a woman's looks.

Being told I was beautiful by a stranger proved I was grown up and out in the world where adventures were possible. *Something was happening.* I dreaded life being boring, life never starting, life only ever happening to other people.

When I was nineteen, did I believe that interesting things never happened to plain women? Quite possibly.

But often the attention came from the wrong men in the wrong way.

Other comments in the 1983 diary:

'I was standing at the bar when some bloke said I had the same face, hair and knockers as Kate Bush...'

'Met a weirdo in the lift who said, "Shame you couldn't stay in here a bit longer..."'

'A man in the town centre said I had lovely long legs...'

'A bloke at the office said he'd overheard a colleague say, "What are Cathy's tits like? Have you felt them yet?"'

It all depended on the intention behind the remarks – and many remarks were threatening, undermining, humiliating and predatory.

Others were said in fun: I was referred to by a friend's mother as 'The Fallen Madonna with the Big Boobies', a reference to a running gag on the sitcom *'Allo 'Allo!*. I pretended not to be embarrassed. Likewise, when a boyfriend's dad often called me 'Sabrina', after a 1950s actress famous for the size of her breasts, I laughed at that, too. I was accustomed to my body being up for judgement, comment and jokes.

The unwanted attention was not only verbal. When I was twenty-three, I was groped in the office by a line manager who grabbed my breasts and squeezed hard during a conversation about tax returns. There was not even the pretence it was anything else – just a brazen lunge and grope as I froze in shock and then tried to stagger backwards to escape.

When I was twenty-five a man shoved his hand between my legs from behind as I queued to get into the Hippodrome theatre in Birmingham to see Ben Elton. There was a big crowd, some jostling, and the unmistakable feeling of being sexually assaulted. I balled my fist, spun round and punched the muscled chest of a big man just behind, as I screamed, 'Don't you fucking touch me!' Furious at being punched, he shouted back – I don't remember what – I can recall only the bits of spit flying out of his mouth, until his laughing friend guided him away.

On another occasion, around the same time, my friend Anita and I were heading off to a New Year fancy dress party – I was wearing an egg-yolk-yellow jacket as Gladys Pugh, a character from the sitcom *Hi-de-Hi!* and Anita was a 'squaw'. We stopped at the motorway services to have a wee and, as I sat there, I saw a man peering over the toilet cubicle to watch me. I have always felt insecure in public toilets and was in the habit of glancing upwards to check as I sat on the loo. This was the first (and only) time I glanced upwards to actually see the top of a face, like a perverted 'Kilroy Was Here' gazing back at me. Anita, trained in arrest and restraint, was in another cubicle. 'Anita, there's a man!' I yelled. Anita valiantly jumped off the loo, yanked down her tassled tunic and kicked the door of the neighbouring cubicle open, but Kilroy had gone.

I reported the office groper to management, I punched the man outside the theatre, I told the police about the voyeur, but these were small fightbacks in a predatory world.

As David Foster Wallace nearly said: That was the water we swam in.

And despite all this, all of the dangers and downsides, I still considered it vital to be considered physically attractive.

I was among a group of young women recruits who did a sketch in the office's 'Christmas Review', which involved wearing swimsuits and glitter and singing a version of 'In the Navy'. There was safety in numbers doing that; it was in public, I was on a 'stage' and the men were not. I was safe there, untouchable. We enjoyed getting a lot of attention from a lot of men who gave a lot of approval. None of us swimsuited dancers considered that we were collaborating in trivialising ourselves at work – nor indeed trivialising any of the other women staff members. We didn't give it a thought – we were having too much fun – high on being young and good-looking in a society that valued youth and good looks in women. It made a dull job more interesting. Anyway, this was an office in which it was considered acceptable to have hard-core porn of women on the walls. I don't think I understood the word 'objectified'. We didn't consider the dancing demeaning; indeed, it gave us a sense of 'power'; an attractive body had become an asset to be shown off, a status symbol. We didn't realise then that youth and looks might end up being the *only* things we were valued for.

On my first day at journalism college, I was sent to do a vox pop – a gathering of opinions from people in the street. My Yes/No questions were: Do you think pictures of topless Page 3 models in newspapers – particularly *The Sun* – encourage sexual harassment? Followed by: Do you think topless Page 3 pictures should be banned? This was the era of glamour model Samantha Fox, one of the most photographed women of the eighties, and it was around this time that MP Clare Short introduced a private members' bill to propose banning Page 3 girls. *The Sun* called her 'Killjoy Clare'.

The answers to my vox pop were yes, a majority thought Page 3 pictures encouraged sexual harassment, and no, they should not be banned. I tried to look polite as I noted down these paradoxical, nonsensical views.

Later, when I worked on a newspaper in the Midlands, day after day I couldn't go out to buy my lunch without being catcalled and harassed by a gang of workmen safely out of reach up a scaffold. *Smile, Love. You don't get many of THEM to the pound.* Jeers, shouts, laughter. I told my male colleagues, but nothing happened until some female members of the public came into the newspaper office to complain that these workmen were in effect making this thoroughfare a no-go area for women. The paper did a story, and I gave them a quote: 'They are animals, they hunt in packs.'

'Come on, Cath!' said my male colleague. 'I can't write that!'

Later still, in my mid-twenties, I started wearing an old suit jacket of my grandad's with the sleeves rolled up – this was a good disguise for big breasts should I need one – until I was at a comedy club and the comedian took it on stage to dangle it from one finger and ridicule it. I got on stage and punched him, too.

Sex and sexuality had been fraught with worry from the shock of puberty, through high school when girls feared falling foul of the social mores and being labelled a 'slut', to the later fear of getting pregnant, of being assaulted, of 'being used', of falling for the wrong man, but in the early eighties the worry took on a new dimension with the arrival of the AIDS epidemic.

First reported in 1981 as affecting gay men in the USA, by 1987 Margaret Thatcher's government had issued an AIDS public information film to be shown during breaks between television programmes.

The actor John Hurt provided the chilling voiceover, to a backdrop of apocalyptic images, crashing music and the tolling of funeral bells: *There is now a danger that has become a threat to us all … It is a deadly disease and there is no known cure …* a volcano erupts, rocks cascade … *the virus can be passed during sexual intercourse with another person … anyone can get it man or woman …* a gravestone is hewn from the rock … *so far it has been confined to small groups, but it is spreading … if you ignore AIDS it could be the death of you* ... the gravestone crashes backwards engraved with the word 'AIDS' ... *so don't die of ignorance...*

It was a forty-second film that stunned the nation. The day after it was first shown, when I was twenty-four years old, I sat in the office with young female colleagues, and we agreed we were terrified. We were making mental checklists of past boyfriends: what if they had had it? What if they didn't know they had it? What if we *already* had it? We could all unknowingly be carrying a deadly, incurable disease.

Leaflets were delivered to every home in the UK recommending the use of condoms for 'safe sex'. Among my peers, contraception was the woman's responsibility. I believed that the pill and tampons were the world's greatest inventions, making it easier to be a woman. The pill was discreet and painless; it was magic – despite the potential side effects of headaches, weight gain, breast pain, blood clots and depression, we thought nothing of taking it year after year. But now we were being asked to bring up the subject of condoms. Despite AIDS being untreatable and fatal, it seemed unthinkable to say the word 'condom' out loud to a man, let alone go and buy some and produce them like a rabbit out of a hat. Unthinkable.

Like I said: my apparent self-confidence was an edifice built on sand.

Never mind 'dying of ignorance', I was more likely to die of embarrassment. When I mentioned to my boss how frightening the film was, he pooh-poohed it. 'We all used to be petrified of TB, and they cured that. Don't worry about AIDS; next year it'll be something else they're worrying about.'

Despite the many pitfalls and dangers of male attention over the years, the need to still be seen as a sexual woman at the age of fifty-four ran deep – indeed it must have been stamped through me like Blackpool rock that not only would my 'value' go down if I lost my femininity, but I would lose a fundamental part of my identity. I felt a deep and creeping fear.

Tamoxifen is an anti-oestrogen treatment that blocks oestrogen activity in my body – and if it is oestrogen that makes us female – what would that make me?

I found myself clicking on a newspaper article entitled 'What is Femininity?' – which felt like a desperate act in itself – only to discover I had opened an advert. The advert blethered on about being 'vibrant, eloquent, charismatic and bold … a new superheroine'. But how was I to achieve this idea of femininity? Apparently, by wearing a perfume called 'Good Girl'. I blinked at it. Where I came from a Good Girl was a child who did as they were told. Or a dog.

I felt angry and frustrated for even having opened the stupid advert.

Flicking through television channels, I caught part of a documentary about tennis player Renée Richards, a trans woman who fought to play on the women's circuit in the 1970s. An interviewee remarked, 'If the doctors have given her the hormones, she's a woman, isn't she?' Which again made me wonder – without the hormones, what was I?

I read a memoir of someone who had transitioned from male to female, who talked about her relief and delight at finally getting access to hormone therapy – to oestrogen – the opposite of what I was going through. She described how her face softened, her breasts developed, she *felt* different. She felt womanly.

I felt bereft.

Kylie Minogue was treated with tamoxifen when she was diagnosed with breast cancer in 2005, so one night as I lay in the sleepless dark, I searched for her on Instagram. I scrolled through images of her in spangly frocks and floor-length dresses, in satin shorts, in a bikini top, jeans and a cowboy hat. Kylie is four years younger than me. Her glamour lit up my bedroom; it didn't matter that she had a team of stylists, hairdressers and beauticians, that the photos must be filtered, that she was a world-famous multimillionaire who was born perfect, because although she may not be relatable in many ways, she was still a middle-aged woman who had had breast cancer, who had gone through hormone treatment and emerged looking womanly, beautiful, happy and living a full life.

I had admired many women in the past but did not remember considering any of them a role model since the horse-riding, school-skipping, monkey-handling Pippi Longstocking. The real-life women of my mother's generation had always seemed too distant from me. Now I did, and I was surprised it was Kylie.

I learned she was due to do a concert in seven months' time at Edinburgh Castle and I decided to be there.

The next morning, back at the hospital, Cello insisted I found someone to talk to about how ill and low I felt.

I explained to a breast care nurse about the side effects of the tamoxifen, the hot flushes, the nausea, the headaches, about the agonising pain down my arm, but as importantly, the mental symptoms. 'I feel hopeless,' I said.

'Hopeless?' she raised her eyebrows and peered at me over her spectacles.

'What is the point?' I said. 'I can't see the point in anything.' She looked surprised, and I blundered on. 'You try to do the right things, but you get cancer anyway. Then you get treatment and that makes things worse.'

'Give it time,' she said, 'it can be hard for women who come here through screening – it's a bolt from the blue because there were no symptoms.'

I blurted out, 'And if there is no oestrogen in my body, I'm frightened I'll turn into a man.'

The nurse and Cello burst out laughing and Cello said, 'You'd have to go some, Cathy.' I started to cry, and the nurse hurriedly stopped smiling and rooted on her shelves for a box of tissues. 'You feel like you're being neutralised?' she asked. 'Well, you're not going to turn into a man.'

A few days later, we visited a friend who was mid-pregnancy and bursting with oestrogen. 'Isn't she glowing?' said Cello. 'She's really glowing, isn't she? She looks amazing!' And I felt myself gulp, before agreeing, that yes, yes, indeed she did.

Twenty-Four

Getting cancer had ripped away any illusion of control and I became obsessed with information gathering. It was vital I found out all I could about cancer, about radiotherapy and about tamoxifen. As always, I was drawn to books and I decided the place I needed to be was the National Library of Scotland.

The National Library is a 'legal deposit library' with the right to claim a copy of every book published in the UK, receiving 5,000 new items every week. This is not a lending library but a mammoth fifteen-storey behemoth of a reference library that disappears into the bowels of the earth behind George IV Bridge in Edinburgh. It contains more than 16 million printed items and has access to millions of other digital records.

I stood and gazed at its austere frontage. Was it art deco or brutalist or a bit of both? I consulted Neil behind the Information desk, who told me the building was begun in 1939 and opened in 1956. He added with a certain perverse pride, 'Sir Nikolaus Pevsner, in his architectural guide of Great Britain, called it "a building of no architectural merit".' We both pondered this. Then Neil added, 'But we've got a hundred and thirty-five miles of shelving,' and we nodded in unison, eyebrows raised. One hundred and thirty-five miles of shelving was *exactly* what I needed.

Even so, I was intimidated by the hushed air of the library, by the wood-panelled, old-volume-lined reading rooms. By the rules and regulations. By the need to have photo ID, but being banned from having pens, only pencils, and no handbags or shopping bags, only see-through carrier bags. I was intimidated by the library's vastness and the sheer amount of information it held.

The library had a copy of the Gutenberg Bible of 1455 and it stored the last letter ever written by Mary Queen of Scots, but it was not these treasures I was after; no, I needed to learn as much as I could about breast cancer and its treatment, about disease and survival, about life and death.

When I walked through the door of the Reading Rooms, I had the sensation of facing an unscalable wall; the place was an impenetrable fortress guarding its vast treasure.

I decided to throw myself at the mercy of the homely-looking woman behind the enquiries desk.

'I want to find out about breast cancer,' I said. She blinked at me. 'Weeell,' she said, 'what in particular?' She had a long-suffering air, as though she had been worn out over the years by the endless procession of would-be researchers who had thrown themselves at her mercy.

'Er...' – how could I say I wanted to know *everything*, I wanted access to *every single thing that had ever been written about breast cancer.*

She tapped on her keyboard and turned the screen to face me. 'So, a search for "Breast Cancer" in our catalogue brings up 393,263 results.' She blinked at me again through her smeary glasses. 'You will have to refine your search.'

Rather than being put off by this, I was delighted. All those books, all those journal entries, those peer-reviewed articles and PhD dissertations. I could hardly wait. I thanked her and found myself a seat at one of the shiny desks with my own screen and keyboard. I glanced around at the other readers: single and silent and studious, deep in their own research. They reminded me of the solitary filmgoers I encountered at the Vue Cinema – all lost in other worlds on this winter's afternoon.

As a fully fledged member of the library, I was armed with my own password through the portal; everything I needed to know about breast cancer was waiting for me there, tantalisingly, at my fingertips, a tap or two away. It was like dipping my toe in the Pacific Ocean – a vast body of water the size of which I could not comprehend, but I was delighted to be able to slip in and begin to slowly, inexpertly, swim without knowing which way I was heading or where I would end up.

I had no system or methodology. I typed in 'Breast Cancer' and up came: *Unveiling the Maelstrom of the Early Breast Cancer Trajectory* and I began to read. Straight away I knew I was in the right place. Here in this academic report was discussion about the 'practical, emotional, relational and existential demands of an illness that intruded every aspect of their lives'. I devoured it and called up another: *Breast Cancer Patients' Experience of External Beam Radiotherapy*; I read that, then another and another. Sometimes the reports were too scientific and complex and were way beyond my understanding, and when that happened it was as though my face was pressed to a window as the glass steamed up, and as hard as I wiped and dodged about, I could not get a clear view.

Sometimes when I didn't understand the reports, when they were about cells and molecules and enzymes, I continued reading anyway because I felt that somewhere within those incomprehensible words was something important to me.

Day after day, when I returned from my radiotherapy session, I headed across the city armed with my notebook and pencil. I read and read. As each afternoon wore on, I kept meaning to go to the library café for a coffee or some sugary shortbread, but there was always another report to read, another article to digest, so I didn't break off but clicked back to the library catalogue to find something else to try to understand. Every afternoon I read until I was dizzy, until the circular domed skylights had turned black and the light an artificial yellow, until my eyes were gritty and a voice crackled over the intercom: *Please note, the library will be shutting in fifteen minutes. Please return all books as soon as possible.* Whereupon I packed my pencil and notebook in my clear carrier bag and stumbled home through the winter dark.

I started this search in the library because 'knowledge is power', because I needed to understand as fully as I could what was happening to me, how and why. But the reading was helping in another way too: the fact that there were many reports and investigations into breast cancer – including early-stage breast cancer – reassured me that it did matter; that it was important to research the impact this disease had on people. This vast body of research and work and thoughts and analysis was an acknowledgement that I have been through something, not nothing.

This seemed obvious to me, but perhaps it was not obvious judging from some comments in the real world.

'Have you put it all behind you now?'

'My mother/sister/grandma had that and she's fine now.'

'Oh, you'll be back to normal in no time.'

These well-intentioned remarks were spoken so emphatically that they acted like gags stopping me from saying what I really thought, which, only three months after diagnosis and while I was still undergoing treatment, was:

'I don't know if I'll ever be able to put this behind me.'

'You may think your mother/sister/grandma is fine now, but have you asked her?'

'What's normal? I'm not sure what that is any more.'

However, instead of saying these things, I would smile and nod, nod and smile. Yes, thank you, fine, thank you. Smile and nod. Anything not to be a nuisance.

Remarks such as these gave me no room to be honest.

Although society no longer shuts down cancer conversations with whispered references to 'The Big C', we shut them down with relentless positivity.

One man cracked a radiotherapy joke: 'You'll be glowing in the dark!' I remembered my Marie Curie Ladybird Book and the gently glowing, dying scientist with her destroyed bone marrow.

Why was this different from Frankie Boyle and his cancer gags that had made me laugh out loud? I think Frankie Boyle had been subverting my fear of cancer – turning it on its head – his jokes were an acknowledgement that cancer was terrifying, but then he added a 'so what? up yours, cancer', plus his jokes weren't aimed at me personally, whereas with milder jokes, to my face, it felt as though the teller was trying to minimise my fear or indeed to deny my right to be fearful at all.

People told me I was being 'brave'. Maybe this was wishful thinking on their part, or maybe they were relieved I wasn't openly sobbing. 'I believe you're being a tough cookie,' one man said, approaching me with his dukes up, fake sparring into thin air.

This idea of cancer being a battle that needs 'fighting' upsets many people because of the implication that those who die did not fight hard enough. I felt that the battle analogy fitted in so far as the doctors were fighting the disease with surgery and radiation and hormone treatment while my body was merely the poor bloody battlefield.

Because how could I 'fight' cancer? If I took on board the 'fighting' idea, it was overwhelming – what if I did not 'fight' it hard enough, or in the right way? I read descriptions of visualisations during which patients were told to picture healthy cells attacking cancerous cells. It was a big responsibility, 'fighting' a disease about which I understood little, with only the power of a visualisation.

There are unwritten rules for cancer patients: be positive, manage your emotions, sanitise your reactions. There is a responsibility not to let this thing get too messy.

Commands I heard often were: 'Be positive', 'Think positive', 'Stay positive' – exhortations to be relentlessly optimistic and courageous. This was often interspersed with other advice: 'Walk every day', 'Juice beets', 'Cut out sugar', 'Don't drink Diet Irn Bru'. But by far the most popular advice was: 'Be positive', 'Think positive', 'Stay positive'.

I was warned about this early on when a friend who had been dealing with cancer for a year wrote to me: 'Everyone told me to be positive and I nearly threw up ... That having to be fucking positive is far more draining than anything else!'

Maybe the idea that cancer patients should be constantly positive is something to say to avoid saying nothing. Or perhaps it means: 'I don't want to hear about your cancer, it makes me too uncomfortable', and we are being prodded into a compliant silence. Or then again, maybe some people really believe that not allowing any sorrow, anger or fear to be expressed will indeed help keep the cancer at bay.

Nevertheless, the idea of fighting the cancer armed with positive thoughts (and its opposite: feeding the cancer with negative thoughts) drips into your consciousness, whether you like it or not, and more than once I found myself desperately spinning in ever-decreasing mind-bending circles: worried that I was worrying because the worry itself may cause the cancer to come back and that made me worry even more, which was worrying because *that* worry may then cause the cancer to come back ... and then it would be MY FAULT that the cancer had come back because I couldn't stop worrying and THAT was very worrying ... and on and on it went, inexorably round and round, further and further down the fear spiral.

Twenty-Four

Some people's idea of 'positive thinking' was the opposite of my fact-finding. A friend told me of an old woman he knew who had survived cancer because she sent her husband back to the library with a flea in his ear when he tried to bring a stack of books about cancer into her house. 'I'm not having those in here!' she apparently declared, ushering her husband and his dangerous books to the door. The person recounting this gave a satisfied nod at this point in the story, as though this tale demonstrated that denying reality was a sure-fire cure for cancer; the indisputable proof was right there in this still-alive old bookless woman and her well-meaning but misguided husband.

I had a vision of all the reports and articles on cancer I had been reading over the preceding days and weeks: 'Er ... that's not really my approach...' and the man shrugged, in a 'don't say I didn't warn you' sort of way and shook his head at the folly of having anything to do with books about cancer, let alone allowing them in the house.

Unsolicited advice is an inevitable hazard of a cancer diagnosis. At a party I was told by someone that exercise was the answer. He told me about a rugby player who exercised his way back to health after cancer treatment. I waited for a gap to tell him I had in fact done four hours of yoga that week, to which he replied, 'Oh ... yoga ... I prefer to actually *do* something.'

Some men acted as though being ill was a competition. 'My wife was much worse than you...' or 'My wife was rushed in for an emergency operation, which trumped her friend's cancer diagnosis...' Sometimes it felt like I was even failing at being ill.

'We all have a bit of cancer in us,' said someone who hadn't been diagnosed with a cancerous tumour.

'Tamoxifen! Oh, that's a miracle drug,' said someone, who didn't have to take it.

Someone else contacted me to point out that the 'birth' of my memoir and the 'releasing of my cancer could not be a coincidence'. This person believed I would make a complete recovery, but the implication seemed to be that if I hadn't written my book I would not have made a complete recovery. It was hard to know exactly.

I read a newspaper article about a woman who was described as 'wearing her cancer as a badge'. Her colleagues got fed up with hearing about her illness. *Is she still going on about it?* The woman was awarded compensation for being driven from her job and 'having her dignity violated'.

Cancer is a hard subject to discuss.

I think back to my friend's text when I told her a potential tumour had been found: '*Fuck! Fuck! Fucking hell! and Fuck! again for good measure.*' And I'm grateful all over again for what a perfect response that was. Not a platitude, not a cliché in sight. And when the physio told me I wasn't 'lucky/unlucky', I was just plain unlucky, it had been a relief to shed the brave face. It had felt good to be seen, and to have the horror of a cancer diagnosis acknowledged rather than minimised.

What a relief it is to be heard and be given the space to be honest.

At the same time, it was hard to *act* honestly. What was a cancer patient supposed to act like? Being so aware that people expect 'bravery' and 'positivity', it was hard to disappoint – who wants to bring the party down? – especially when you have been raised not to be a nuisance, to be cooperative, to smile and be nice.

Early in the radiotherapy I was invited to the Scottish Parliament to celebrate the work of the Scottish Book Trust. I was asked to read an excerpt from my memoir due for publication three months later. This was the first time I had read from the book in public and I had an actual copy of the book in my hands – a proof copy, but still a copy. It was a big moment, but I was not sure what to do with my face. I have a Resting Bitch Face – a face that falls into an unfriendly deadpan expression when I may be feeling no emotion at all.

I didn't know the phrase 'Resting Bitch Face' when I was growing up, but I became aware as a child that something about me prompted men to goad me. *Smile, it might never 'appen.* I would be jolted out of private thoughts and daydreams, *Cheer up, Love, world 'asn't ended,* and I'd feel embarrassed that *somehow,* I had got it wrong and caused offence.

As a child I was surprised that the act of *being* attracted any attention at all, let alone what felt like barely disguised hostility. Did everyone get this reaction, or was it only me? What was my face doing, when I took my mind off it, that provoked and challenged people? Did I not look happy enough, attentive enough, present, approachable, open enough? Was I too unfriendly, sullen, miserable, selfish? Was I not giving them something I owed – smiles, attention, interest? Their remarks seemed to demand a response, an apology perhaps, I was not sure, but I felt criticised and humiliated.

My facial expression became another thing to make me self-conscious.

Years later I mentioned the phenomenon of being told to smile by strangers in the street to an older male acquaintance. He assured me he had never done it, indeed he had neither seen it nor heard of it being done and what was more he had checked, and it had never happened to his wife either, that, in fact, he found it hard to believe it happened at all.

On my wedding day, aged thirty, I was frightened that my Resting Bitch Face would ruin the photographs. How could I banish Resting Bitch Face for the day? I practised a half-smile as though that was how my face fell naturally – but it looked decidedly unnatural.

Maybe if I repeated the thought *Everything is Perfect* it would show on my face? I decided to try this – as I was walking down the aisle, as I was sitting at the top table, as I was eating, drinking, waiting, listening, I diligently wore my mask. *Everything is Perfect. Everything is Perfect.*

It was a lot of effort to look normal.

Now, at the Scottish Parliament, I was again adjusting my mask. It was a complicated expression to calculate. I was having a book published (big smile, grateful and happy – but not smug); the book was about the death by suicide of my sister (no smile at all); I was in the middle of cancer treatment, during which I was apparently being 'brave' and 'positive' (stoic, rather wry smile).

I Googled: 'How to get rid of Resting Bitch Face' and found: 'Wear eyeliner, engage cheeks, look up.' Another article said medical professionals were happy to 'battle' Resting Bitch Face by injecting fillers and Botox. Apparently, to stop women looking 'off-putting' or a 'sourpuss' and risking 'giving a first date the wrong impression', the doctors could 'correct' the woman's expression, giving them 'a more pleasant pout', which would 'literally turn your frown upside-down!' It was almost a relief that they were offering to inject and freeze smiles on our faces and not to permanently stitch a smile on.

At the parliament, I gave myself confidence by wearing high heels (mostly abandoned these days in favour of comfort and speed in trainers). I came through the airport-style security with a bag of shoes and hopped from foot to foot, changing them in the entranceway before arriving in the main foyer four inches taller.

One of the first people I saw was another writer who was treated for breast cancer ten years ago. We were mainly friends through Facebook rather than real life – but I wanted to cling to her like a life raft. 'How are you?' she asked, and the question was genuine and full of understanding. I blurted out about the tamoxifen nightmare and she replied, 'Bloody tamoxifen! The side effects are never a glorious mane of hair and the arse of a goddess, are they?' We laughed a genuine laugh of shared experience and it was a wonderful relief.

Another writer approached to find out what was so funny and when we said, 'We're talking about being treated for breast cancer', she raised her hands and backed off as though she was intruding at a wake. 'It's okay,' we said, 'do come and join in.'

For the reading I had edited together a short piece about my love of books to fit the occasion. *As a child, books were my escape from a world with the wrong kind of drama in it. I hungered for stories to make reality fall away ... I read to find circuses, wild animals, long dresses, and magic faraway trees ... I read the back of the cereal packet ... the primary school library over and over again ... the set texts my big sister brought home from secondary school. I read the* Daily Express *... the* Radio Times *... I read the dictionary.*

It made me realise I hadn't changed much. Nowadays it was reports about cancer in the Scottish National Library, but I had always needed access to the other people's words; to their ideas, their worldviews, their brains, their learning, to entertain and educate me, to help me escape, to help me get through this life in this body.

The radiotherapy days ticked by. I read an account by a radiotherapy patient in the US in which she mentioned having a warm blanket placed on her body during the treatment. A warm blanket!? Not a crepe paper 'cover cloth' quivering in the cold draft from the air conditioning? I took a fluffy cardigan into the treatment room and asked if they could place it on my body once they had positioned me to keep me warm. Yes, no problem, they said, and I was flabbergasted. Why had they left me to freeze for nearly three weeks, with my hypermobile shoulders reacting to the cold, when I could have had my cardigan on top of me to keep me warm?

One day my session was scheduled for late in the day. It was different being in the Cancer Centre late afternoon when it had gone dark outside, the hustle and bustle had quietened and the crowds inside had thinned. There was the crash of the shutters as the WRVS coffee bar closed; the calls of the staff – *Bye!* – and the screech of the sliding doors as they headed home; the cries of an exhausted child face down emitting a relentless wail on one of the waiting-room sofas. The dying of a day. A sense of an ending, and I was so relieved to pass though those sliding doors myself and escape into the dark.

Kindness and care came from unexpected sources. It was mid-winter and our central heating broke down. We were struggling to fit the gasman in around my hospital appointments, which, usually being around noon, wrote off the whole day for the provider. The gas engineer who eventually arrived was baffled by our old boiler. He clanged around for a while to no avail. I was wrapped in a blanket on the sofa when I heard him yelling down his phone in the hall, 'This woman's got cancer! I've got to get this boiler working. This woman's got cancer!'

The following day a Polish roofer arrived for a routine roof inspection. We left him to it and shot off to the hospital. On our return, he took Cello aside and said he was going to pray for me at his Friday night prayer group.

Two weeks into the radiotherapy I had a slow-crawling sensation in my sinuses. It was not quite dizziness, not quite sickness, not quite confusion. It was impossible to know if this was the radio-therapy, the tamoxifen, the sleeplessness, the stress of the whole situation or a toxic cocktail of everything. Then I saw the first review of *When I Had a Little Sister*. It was unexpected, months before publication. The review described the book as 'brave' and 'elegiac' (a word that made me reach for my *Oxford Paperback Dictionary*). I experienced a rush of delight that made my scalp prickle, followed by a breathtaking horror that my family's story was now public.

The fear of the book's publication mingled with the fear of the cancer and it was hard to separate them – the 'dream come true' and the 'nightmare' creating a knot in my stomach and a swirling fear in which one was indistinguishable from the other.

I knew I needed help with my anxiety, and someone suggested going to Maggie's Edinburgh, a drop-in centre based at the Western for anyone affected by cancer. I half-wondered if going to Maggie's was embracing cancer a bit too much – but that was an excuse because I was intimidated at the thought of it.

I put my name down for 'Drop-in Relaxation'. The centre was light-filled, brightly decorated, and had lots of niches with armchairs and soft blankets. There was a central table with a full fruit bowl, plates of biscuits and 'Margaret's cheese scones'.

I squeezed in around the table beside a lady with a broad Lancashire accent and helped myself to a Jammie Dodger. I told her it was my first visit and she said she had only started coming twelve months after her treatment finished when everyone thought she should have 'got over it'.

I told her I was on tamoxifen and she muttered 'poor you', and we both munched our biscuits. For a second, we morphed into Les Dawson and Roy Barraclough's Cissie and Ada, and I half-expected one of us to adjust a bosom and declare we were a slave to our hormones.

'You could put some money in the pot for the Monday Club,' she said. 'We buy Cup-a-Soups.' I thanked her. I was not sure I wanted to be a member of the Monday Club with their Cup-a-Soups; most of the people looked twenty years older than me and one man kept talking about the 'device' he needed to pee. For a moment I wondered if me and the Lancashire lady had blundered into the prostate cancer support group.

I heard other snatches of conversation: ...*I'm asking if I can go to Australia ... I'm having my bloods done ... It's a change of life-style ... I know there's no guarantees, of course there's not ... I had the camera treatment, but it wasn't flexible ... If anything went wrong it'd be a blue light up to the Royal ... How can I use that to pee when I already need two sticks?*

Someone appeared, balancing a birthday cake on a plate on outstretched palms with the candles lit, and a raggle-taggle of voices broke out into *Happy Birthday to you, Happy Birthday to you, Happy Birthday dear...* nobody seemed sure, but we picked up again for a resounding finale: *Happy Birthday to you!*

On the table, among the birthday cake and biscuits, lay leaflets: *Writing Your Will, Power of Attorney, Living Wills, Inheritance Tax.*

We went to a separate room for the relaxation class; yet more comfortable sofas and armchairs and a view of a kinetic sculpture in the garden, which twisted elegantly in the breeze.

We closed our eyes, and the class leader took us through a talking meditation, a guided visualisation. She had a gentle, comforting voice that lulled and beguiled. *You are barefoot on a sandy beach ... you are paddling in the sea ... you write a word in the sand, it says 'living'...*

There were renovations going on in the garden and from outside we heard the odd clang of a hammer and scrape of a spade, while inside there was gentle snoring from one of the drop-in relaxers who had dropped off. I felt deeply relaxed; I was both in the room and not in the room, on the sofa and on a sandy beach, aware of my surroundings and yet somewhere else.

After the class I discovered that Maggie's also had a library. It was built around a gurgling tank of electric-blue fish flitting among artificial plants. My eyes skimmed the shelves – so many different cancers, so many different stories. *You & Leukaemia, Your Guide to Bowel Cancer, Living with a Brain Tumour.* Despite the subject matter, I found myself thrilling to the idea of another library, another body of books at my disposal. There were chatty, informal testimonies from people who have lived through it: *No More Bad-Hair Days, It's Not Like That Actually.* There were spiritual ones: *Beyond Miracles, The Anatomy of Hope, The Mindful Path to Self-Compassion.* At the top was a large section on diet: *The Allergy Bible, Eat for Immunity, The Soft Diet.* And at the bottom: *Guiding Your Child Through Grief, What Happened to Daddy's Body?, What Does Dead Mean?*

Twenty-Five

As a teenager my skin was so white it was blue-white. The first time I stood on a beach in a bikini I was twenty-two years old, and my friend, Anita, said, 'I have never seen anyone as white as you.' We were in Malia, Crete, for a fortnight to escape real life. We had set great store by this holiday; this was a new beginning. We had spent many evenings in Mario's Italian restaurant discussing how this holiday would change our lives. We were going to come back *different people*. And the first and most important step in becoming different people was to get a tan.

This was 1986 and tans were BIG. They were also dark, deep, fast, rich and sexy, according to some suntan lotion ads, or tropical, wild and savage, according to others. Ads urged sunbathers to 'stay just a little bit longer', mocking those who cowered under hats and umbrellas.

Tans were San Tropez and yachts; they were California and surfing; they were *Dynasty* and *Dallas*; they were glamour and sophistication; tans were *slimming*.

We did not know that tans became desirable only after Coco Chanel got one in the 1920s, and had previously been associated with outdoor farm labourers and looked down upon. And nor would we have cared.

I had tried unsuccessfully to get a tan by visiting sunbeds, but after almost fusing my contact lenses to my eyeballs, I had been put off.

Unfortunately, on our first day in Crete, a wind whipped up the deserted beach, sandblasting us as we lay on our brand new beach towels, gazing at the overcast sky. 'Perhaps it's so hot we can't feel it,' one of us suggested hopefully. When it began to rain, we grabbed our towels, beach bags, flip-flops and hats and retreated despondent to the nearest taverna, listening to the splattering drops on the thatched roof.

'And the weather's been so great for weeks,' said the barman.

The next day the sun shone, and for the rest of the holiday getting a tan became a cross between a scientific experiment and a full-time job.

Let's get in the sun and flog it!

First, we worked on our 'base tans', suffering through various burn/peel cycles on different parts of the body – back of the neck, shoulders, inside the ankles, top of the feet. We removed everything bar bikini bottoms to avoid tan lines; gone was the last vestige of my self-consciousness about having big breasts. I got Anita to take a photograph to prove it – a photograph I realised years later had been pilfered from my photo album.

We turned ourselves regularly to ensure the front matched the back, applying dabs of sun protection factor 8 'to be on the safe side', excitedly waiting for the tan to 'turn' from red to brown. Every evening we examined ourselves in the full-length mirrors. *Has my tan turned?* Gawping over our shoulders, watching our buttocks get more startlingly white and uncooked as the holiday progressed, admiring how flashing-white our eyes and teeth looked. We went out wearing white to show off the tan, we wore off-the-shoulder clothing to show off the tan.

It was agony lathering aftersun lotion on tender burns, legs twitching with stabbing pains, skin on fire all night long under sheets that felt too heavy. Sunburn is a pain that lingers in my memory, but we still went back to offer ourselves to the sun gods all over again the next day. No talk of skin cancer, melanoma or skin damage in 1986, not even a mention of wrinkles.

And it wasn't only the women; the men were as keen to be brown, and many had entire backs burnt red-raw.

The second week was all about 'deepening' the tan in the vain hope it would last more than a week once we got home. No suntan lotion was used at this stage – just a glistening layer of Johnson's Baby Oil, as we stretched out, greasy and hot as rotisserie chickens, to a backdrop of 'When the Going Gets Tough'.

Nothing else was as important – certainly not the Club 18-30 games taking place on the beach nearby, including 'Pass the Cucumber', where participants rolled onto each other passing a cucumber groin to groin down a long line, man to woman, as Frankie said 'Relax'.

I lay in the sun reading the Jilly Cooper bonkbuster *Riders*, trying to make sure the 900-odd pages didn't cast a shadow on my face. *Sex and horses: who could ask for more?* yelled the blurb on the back of the book. I devoured details of the anti-hero Rupert Campbell-Black, the 'promiscuous upper-class cad' with his 'denim blue eyes' and 'haughty suntanned features', to the sound of women shrieking as mechanics and forklift truck drivers from Milton Keynes thrust cucumbers between their legs. Rupert Campbell-Black they were not. No life imitating art here.

Anita and I had left Manchester Airport two weeks before in our matching turquoise ski pants and yellow T-shirts, with so much fluorescent holiday wear we could barely shut our suitcases, and with our hopes sky high. We returned home the same people – except the colour of mahogany wardrobes. When I went back to work my boss said, 'By 'eck, Cath, I think you've overdone that a bit.'

My daughters are from a generation where tans are equally desirable, but they have been taught to 'fake not bake'. When I tell them about the great Cretan tan of 86, Lara asks if I wasn't afraid of 'blackfishing'. I have never heard the term and she explains that blackfishing is a white person taking on physical aspects of a black person – hair, skin colour – a practice that is considered a form of cultural appropriation.

1986 seems like a very long time ago.

By the end of the radiotherapy, the skin on my breast and torso was burnt and sore despite all the faithful application of creams. The fold under my breast felt so tender I hardly dared to touch it in case it blistered and broke open like an over-ripe fruit. I dried it by dabbing once or twice with a towel, holding my breath in case the skin split. At the suggestion of the radiotherapists, I had been wearing cotton hankies against my skin to protect it for the past two weeks. I had found an old handkerchief of my dad's, so not only was I wearing a granny bra, but there was a ruffle sticking out all around with *Present from the Isle of Man* embroidered on it.

On my final day, I snapped photos of my surroundings as I walked down the Cancer Centre corridor. I needed to take away bits of this place to come to terms with my time here. I took pictures of the side room with three blue armchairs arranged round a coffee table containing only a box of tissues with the next tissue poking out, poised, waiting. I took a picture of oxygen tanks attached to trolleys lined up in the corridor like wallflowers at a disco.

In an odd way this place had become comforting as it became familiar.

'It's your last day,' trilled the receptionist and it did feel significant. In some places they sound a gong to mark the ending of hospital treatment, but not here.

I went through the rigmarole of the treatment for the last time, and afterwards I clambered off the bed and went behind the curtain to get dressed. Balanced on top of my bra and *Present from the Isle of Man* cotton hankie was a leaflet: *After Radiotherapy: What Now?*

Twenty-Five

When I emerged from the cubicle into the cold room everyone else had gone.

I was warned that the effects of the radiotherapy would peak two weeks after finishing and I inspected my skin every day – hardly daring to look. It became increasingly burnt and it was alarming to watch it worsen day by day, even after the hospital visits had finished. There were stabbing and shooting pains in my breast and I found myself reading, eating or working at my computer wincing and clutching my breast to lessen the pain. I had to stop myself doing this in public, or at least make sure I did it under my coat.

I went for a walk because fresh air on my face improved my mood. In a book shop I found a copy of *Werner's Nomenclature of Colours with Additions*. This was a book originally published in 1812 to describe colours by finding examples of where they appeared in nature, in animal, vegetable or mineral form. A copy was taken by Charles Darwin on his travels. I browsed the book and because everything in my mind linked back to cancer and my constant internal monologue about it, I looked in it for all the shades of red, purple, pink and brown currently manifesting themselves on my breast.

According to *Werner's Nomenclature of Colours*, my right armpit was 'Auricula Purple' (the same colour as the *Egg of Largest Blue Bottle or Flesh Fly*) mixed with 'Deep Reddish Brown' (*Neck of Teal Drake* or *Dead Leaves of Green Panic Grass*) alongside touches of 'Hair Brown' (*Head of a Pintail Duck*) with raw, freshly peeled areas of 'Flesh Red' (*Larkspur*). The main part of the breast was 'Vermillion Red' (*Red Coral* or *Love Apple*) and 'Carmine Red' (*Cock's Comb*), while the underside of the breast was a riot of 'Scarlet Red' (*Mark on the Head of the Red Grouse*), 'Purplish Red' (*Precious Garnet*), 'Cochineal Red' (*Underside of Decayed Leaves* of None-so-Pretty), 'Brownish Purple Red' (*Flower of Deadly Nightshade*), 'Pansy Purple' (*Sweet-Scented Violet*) and 'Clove Brown' (*Head and Neck of a Male Kestrel*).

The book's introduction said it was 'highly useful to the Arts and Sciences, particularly … Morbid Anatomy', and I wondered how many other people had used it to describe their radiation burns.

My burnt breast was an alarming sight, and I felt a certain satisfaction when I went to Lara's bedroom later, in my dressing gown, to show her and she recoiled with a shriek.

Twenty-Six

Two weeks after the radiotherapy finished, the fatigue was intense. My head and body were full of cement. I was exhausted to my finger-ends – every atom – but resting on the bed did not ease the fatigue. I crawled upstairs on all fours and showered leaning against the tiles. I felt a desire to lie down even as I was already lying down. I wanted to sink into the bed, through the bed and keep on sinking until I felt the centre of the earth take the weight of my body and allow me to rest.

The immediate hospital treatment was completed, and I would return for a check-up in six weeks. The *After Radiotherapy: What Now?* leaflet warned that finishing treatment could be an emotional time because there was 'reduced contact with the hospital and people can feel isolated and low'. 'Please do not hesitate to seek advice and support at this time,' it said.

But what advice? From whom? I couldn't imagine what anyone could do or say. All of the literature warned about radiotherapy fatigue – defining fatigue as 'a tiredness that cannot be assuaged by rest'.

There was no miracle cure.

Yet still I contrived to take part in the charade of 'bouncing back'.

I attended a friend's book launch, plastered in make-up, my face highlighted to a brilliant sheen. 'You're glowing!' people said, and we chinked glasses and I replied, 'Radiotherapy's over – I've turned a corner!' I kept up this performance for two hours. By the time I got home, I was so exhausted I wanted to weep.

Why did I pretend to feel better? Partly because I wanted it to be true, and partly because I was frightened of boring people.

I went upstairs to lie down and discovered the skin peeling off my entire right breast –including my nipple – something I didn't even know could happen.

As I lay on the bed thinking there was nothing to be done but wait it out, my publisher emailed the final cover for my memoir and suddenly, although my body was sore and leaden, my heart was singing.

From despair to elation in a moment.

I was a guest at the Saltire Society Literary Awards. Hundreds of us filled Dynamic Earth, which was lit up pink and purple with stars projected on the ceiling, circling among the festoons of fairy lights and dangling snowflakes. I sat by the door on the first chair I came to.

I was literally and emotionally on the periphery of this event.

On the opposite side of the round table were two well-known writers – an Edinburgh doctor who has written a book about the body, which included a chapter on breast cancer, and a poet who has written about her personal experience of breast cancer. The music was loud; it was possible to talk only to those directly beside me, but I had a momentary urge to dash around the table and throw myself upon the mercies of the doctor and the poet, these experts on breast cancer, and beg for reassurance. With their magical capabilities with medicine and words, they could surely divulge whatever it was I needed to know on how to start living again.

But I did not. Instead, I gulped my prosecco and ate a biscuit with 'Saltire Literary' iced on top.

The winner of The Saltire Book of the Year was a popular choice with the crowd: it was *All That Remains: A Life in Death*, by Sue Black – the book that discussed the wisdom of medical screening, which Cello had read out to me when I was wondering whether to go for my mammogram six months ago.

I felt lonely and disconnected from my surroundings.

My body was aching from top to bottom and my bones were getting heavier and heavier. I knew I must leave before I became incapable of getting off the chair. An announcement was made that the bar was now open and everyone was encouraged to mingle.

Instead, I headed to the cloakroom where, feeling like Cinderella, I swapped my high heels for trainers.

I came to writing late – only starting aged forty-five. I knew no one in the writing world and I recall the first time I attempted 'networking'– a word that terrified me until I realised it meant 'chatting'. My friend Frances and I went to our first networking event together. We stood at the bar drinking two orange juices, our backs to the room, speaking to no one, before fleeing into the night. I have got better at networking since then, and before cancer I would have loved this event.

I resented cancer forcing me away and wresting this evening from my grasp, but I didn't have the strength to argue.

I slipped out. From across the road I could hear the music booming as the brightly lit building glowed like something from another planet.

I became frightened of trying to sleep. I used to love my duvet – it was so welcoming – yet now, at the end of another sleepless night, when I had fought a constant battle with it and neither of us had won, it felt like the enemy. My bed was a battleground of rumpled sheets and burning pillows.

It used to be babies that kept me awake at night. I remembered the heavy loneliness of night-time feeds. I remembered gazing over neighbouring rooftops searching for any lit windows, wondering who else was awake at this other-worldly hour, who else was sharing this dark stillness. I remembered feeling the warmth of the baby's head against my cheek as I rocked her back to sleep trying not to feel disconnected from a world that motherhood had thrown me out of.

Now, in a different house, and a different time, I stared up at Calton Hill, at the linked pools of light on the path to the top, and I was again disconnected from the world, but now there was no quietness, no stillness, as my skin burned and my thoughts rampaged, creating chaos in mind and body.

I dreaded sleeplessness and delayed going to bed. Perhaps it was easier not to try to sleep at all. Instead, I dropped off on the sofa for a few minutes at a time, the television forcing its way into my consciousness like an assault, blaring its way around my brain and prodding me awake with the shock of the adverts.

Often, I saw every hour and counted the sleep I got in minutes. I lay uncovered on a December night, my skin prickling with heat. Frightening thoughts circled, repeating over and over: *What's the point? There's no point!* And yet I knew there was a point, I must have done, because I was filled with terror that the cancer would come back and kill me. But that didn't stop the thoughts: *What's the point? There's no point!*

I was tempted to lie down on the cold bathroom tiles, but I knew the chills would set in straight away and I might never stop shivering, even as I burned. I had never realised it was possible to be hot and cold at the same time.

Days and nights merged as I lay in despair through the silent hours waiting for the first unwelcome chinks of sunrise and, despite my burning skin, I knew why they called it the 'cold' light of day. Sometimes I fell into a surface-sleep just before the alarm rang and I jolted awake with a frisson, a heavy head and gritty eyes, and it was like the pennies were already weighing down my eyelids.

We went to see *Macbeth*, and when he cried, 'Sleep no more, Macbeth doth Murder sleep,' I almost shouted back, 'Yes!'

How unbearable it is to live without restful sleep.

I sought salvation back at the National Library of Scotland. I went to the Special Collections Room on the fifteenth floor where they store the manuscripts published before 1851 and asked to see 'Night Thoughts' by Edward Young. In this poem, Young describes his insomnia, opening with a description of what he desires most: 'Tired Nature's sweet restorer, balmy sleep.' He goes on: 'Silence and darkness! Solemn Sisters,' and I nodded, solemn sisters, indeed.

There was something moving, and quite electrifying in reading obsessive night thoughts written in the 1740s by a man facing up to life, death and mortality; thoughts written in a poetic language of 250 years ago but with which I could wholly identify.

I carefully turned the thick pages in this version dating from 1797 as it lay in its protective wooden cradle, held in place by weighted cords. To my left was a floor-to-ceiling glass wall with a view over the grey roofs and domes of Edinburgh to the Lion Hill of Arthur's Seat. There were only three other readers. The room was hushed, just the hum of the air conditioning, the clearing of a throat, the turning of a page. It was Christmas week, the week of the shortest day, and by mid-afternoon the sky had turned a deep indigo.

I switched on my lamp and continued to read.

Young lamented the passing of time and how we do not appreciate it until it is too late. 'Time is dealt out by particles ... Where is tomorrow? – in another world!' And in the most well-known lines from the poem: 'Procrastination is the thief of time. Year after year it steals, till all are fled.'

He warned: 'All mankind mistake their time of day,' and talked of 'The disappointment of a promised hour.'

I was reminded of my mother, who said on her seventieth birthday – a year after her initial cancer diagnosis – that she had received her 'three score years and ten' promised in the Bible and could ask for no more. Yet on her deathbed, five years later, as she forced down her now-pointless medication, the non-Hodgkins lymphoma having almost got the better of her organs, she said to Cello, 'I would do anything for another day.'

Young writes: 'Man feels a thousand deaths in fearing one.'

As with the pork pie-munching Wittgenstein at the cinema, I felt such kinship with him.

On a visit to the British Library in London I saw a copy of 'Insomniac' by Sylvia Plath, handwritten and covered in crossings-out, in which she wrote about thoughts repeating 'over and over' as 'memories jostle' in the 'blueblack' night. Plath wrote this poem about the frenzied, distorted, hysterical thoughts of an insomniac in 1961 and it won a prize at the Cheltenham Literary Festival. In a letter displayed alongside the manuscript, she wrote: 'I am very happy ... that sleeplessness has its own very pleasant reward.'

I believed the poem.

I did not believe the letter. She was being polite. There is no reward – not even literary prizes – that are worth the agony of sleeplessness.

Was it odd that I felt more connection with Young, a poet dead for two hundred years, than some of my contemporaries?

A friend wrote saying he believed illness was symbolic of deeper truths and suggested that breast cancer arose from a lack of self-nurture and self-acceptance.

I gazed at the message, taken aback, lost for words. I paced the house going hot and cold, and then replied in a more measured tone than I felt, saying I disagreed with what he said as it slithered down the slippery slope of blaming patients for their illnesses.

Yes, yes, of course, came back the reply that is not what was meant at all.

I was still upset by the message hours later when I told Nina about it.

She raised her eyebrows. 'What people say is about them not about you,' she said. 'They comfort themselves with the idea that by doing everything right they can control their chance of getting cancer – you have failed, but they tell themselves, they will not.'

I was reminded of how many times I had asked 'Do they smoke?' when I'd heard about cancer diagnoses. When we hear about cancer, our thoughts are for ourselves, how we differ from the cancerous person, how cancer happened to them and not us, how we are protected from their fate.

A private message arrived on Facebook asking me to post pink hearts to all my friends for Breast Cancer Awareness.

Didn't me having breast cancer and telling my friends about it already raise awareness? What further good would a pink heart do? What information would it impart?

What if I, or anyone else with breast cancer, had momentarily forgotten we had breast cancer – as if! – maybe we didn't want reminding with messages about pink hearts.

Maybe we had had all the awareness we could stand.

Cancer was everywhere, bombarding me from all angles.

I received an email with the subject line: I AM SUFFERING FROM CANCER OF THE HEART.

Dear Friend. Greetings to you in the name of the Lord God Almighty. I am MRS RUKIA NIMINE from (Paris) France… I have been suffering from this deadly disease called cancer for long and the doctor just said I have just few days to leave… Now, that I am about to end the race like this, without any family members and no child… I have $5.8

One Body

Million US DOLLARS in BANK OF AFRICA, Burkina Faso its all my life savings… Mrs Rukia Nimine went on to say she would give me half of her $5.8 Million US DOLLARS if I promised to give the other half to an orphanage of my choice.

I resented Mrs Rukia Nimine, not because she was trying to scam me but because she sent me scurrying to Google, to search 'Cancer of the Heart'.

I was having lunch with friends when one asked another, 'Any luck with that bloke from work?' and when I enquired who this would-be boyfriend was, the answer came: 'His wife died of cancer', and the food turned tasteless in my mouth.

When you have been forced to face your own mortality, hearing stories about 'moving on' after a bereavement are shocking – you imagine it is you they are moving on from, you who has been left behind, marooned, as others walk away into a distance you will never see.

I felt so old. Cancer had aged me twenty years. I ached, I forgot, I needed to keep lying down, I could not see beyond ill-health. I went to the People's Palace, a museum in Glasgow, with Lara and we wandered around the eccentric exhibits – Billy Connolly's banana boots, Rab C. Nesbit's vest – and I stumbled upon a glass case about 'old age' that contained corsets, suspenders and false teeth. Looking at these sad artefacts representing ageing sent a shock through me, like prodding a sore tooth.

I was blurry-minded and confused. Again, I didn't know if this was the radiotherapy, the insomnia, the tamoxifen or the stress, or most likely a combination of everything. My head and body were full of lead. My brain was full of white noise, like the interference on our childhood television set.

Twenty-Six

I tried to help by making lists, but by the time I had picked up my pen I had forgotten what I meant to write. I went into rooms to find half-finished jobs; messages written and not sent; ingredients spread on the worktop but not assembled into a meal; the oven on with nothing in it; notes jotted down in my handwriting that made no sense. When I found myself arriving in a room unaware why, I would retrace my steps, trying to locate the moment my memory vanished.

I felt distanced from reality as though I was encased in a glass box. The week before Christmas I went to the hairdresser's and as she wrapped me in the nylon robe, I had a flashback to the hospital gown.

In the salon there were Lindor chocolates the colour of Santa's suit, heavy glossy magazines: *What the Vogue Editors are wearing for New Year's Eve!* There was a lively playlist: *It's Chrisssst-masssss!* There was frothy coffee and cinnamon biscuits in the shape of Christmas trees, but I was trapped behind the plate glass. I was bodily in the hairdresser's; I could see it, feel it, taste it, hear it and smell it but I could not live it.

I confided in a friend a few years older than me, who replied, 'Oh, I'm like that, that's just getting old.' In response to my silence she then added, 'Not that I'm minimising the way you are feeling or anything.'

I was fifty-four when I was diagnosed, I was now fifty-five – the age my mother was when she went through the menopause. I imagined how much worse this whole cancer nightmare must be for younger women plunged into these symptoms in their twenties, thirties and forties. How robbed they must feel.

Someone said to me, 'People get cancer much younger than you, you know', as though I didn't know, as though my heart didn't clench whenever I walked past the unbearable sign for the Teenage Cancer Centre in the hospital.

I went back to Maggie's for another guided relaxation. I was in 'my place' on the sofa. I had only been once before but as a creature of habit this spot was 'my place'. I had already had my Jammie Dodger.

It was the same leader with her musical voice: *You are walking through the woods ... you are sitting with your back against a tree...* I kept my eyes clenched shut and tried to concentrate. *Your feet are on the cool wet grass...* Maybe it was the phrase 'cool wet grass', I don't know, but today my mind would not do this. Reality kept barging in. *Your toes are in the water...* No, today my toes were definitely not in the water. I lost concentration, letting go of the visualisation like a deflating balloon, and I fumed: what did I do to deserve this?

Christmas was pared down; that was one good thing about cancer. I don't know why I needed an excuse not to write cards, not to buy and wrap unwanted presents, not to overdecorate the house, overbuy food, book nights out I didn't want, but it seems I did.

I played carols and lit candles and enjoyed knowing Christmas would arrive on the 25th and be gone by the 26th regardless. Lara and I indulged in what has become a family tradition: 'Sherry and Perry' – a glass of Harveys Bristol Cream with Perry Como's 'Here We Come a-Caroling' crackling away on the turntable.

I found an email I wrote to a friend ten years ago, shortly after breaking my arm in the run-up to Christmas. In it I had written, 'Fortunately I had just finished all the Christmas shopping and wrapping that day, so my timing wasn't bad.'

I begged to differ with my old self – my timing was terrible. Fancy having a broken arm and *still* not escaping Christmas.

A friend, Rita, asked if she could treat me to a 'gong bath' by her daughter, Melissa, who was a sound therapist. I had never heard of such a thing and imagined myself scratching about in a great bird bath.

I had realised by now that cancer brought many new experiences – some of which were good: Britney, red lipstick, guided visualisations, pared-down Christmases and now, apparently, gong baths.

I drove out to Rita's home in the countryside not sure what to expect from this new 'cancer experience'.

I lay on a treatment bed, in the best sitting room. The curtains were drawn, and I was covered in silky and fleecy blankets. I shut my eyes as Melissa moved around the room repeating mantras in Sanskrit, making noises with shakers and 'singing bowls' and low-rumbling gongs that built up to dramatic crescendos – gongs so big I could feel the draught when they moved.

At first, I was self-conscious; it was hard to forget I was lying on a bed in a friend's house in the middle of the day as her daughter shook shakers, banged gongs and chanted. But once I was over that, I found the experience strangely affecting. The sound was inside me; every cell in my body seemed to respond, as though I had become an instrument myself. It reminded me of the out of body experience of being under hypnosis.

Afterwards I explained that I had felt an overwhelming sensation moving through my body and Rita said, 'Oh! You had an energy orgasm', and I marvelled that truly there was no end to this cancer experience.

Twenty-Seven

Months earlier the doctor had said it would be a good idea to have something to look forward to after the treatment.

I wanted to book a trip and worried I would not get travel insurance, but our insurers said I was covered for everything not cancer-related.

We went to see Faisal, our travel agent, who was busy booking a pilgrim's visit to Mecca. As we waited, I gazed about the tiny shop at the brochure displays with names like *Intrepid, Mountain Heights* and *Incredible Journeys*. They sounded like hard work.

I studied a map of the world that half-filled the wall. Before I got cancer, I had dreamed of visiting Buenos Aires. I found the city on Faisal's map, and was taken aback by how far it seemed now, how remote, how distant from doctors and safety. Seven thousand miles across the Northern and Southern Atlantic Ocean – I may as well be blasted off into outer space. Would I ever be brave enough to plan such a thing now that my world had changed?

Cancer had shrunk my life.

We asked Faisal where we could fly directly from Edinburgh on 27 December, for a week. He suggested going to Valencia for a few days, then taking the train to Barcelona and flying home from there.

I was nervous about the energy it would take, but we could take our time. Rest often.

We booked it, and the tickets had become a talisman drawing me through the treatment.

Which was how I found myself at New Year in the most beautiful place I had ever been. The midday sun steamed blood-red, gold, green and blue through the stained-glass windows of the Sagrada

Família in Barcelona. The sunbeams coloured the air and painted the walls, the floor and the pillars, which soared up to a heaven I didn't even believe in.

Except here, for a moment, maybe I did.

The red was redder, the blue was bluer, the green so green I wanted to dance in it. I stood, head back, neck craning, immersed in the magnitude of Gaudí's masterpiece, trying to keep the moment intact.

I took photographs, but they were not enough; they were not big enough, deep enough or magnificent enough. No matter how many I took, or how I angled the camera or zoomed in or out, the results did not do justice to this wondrous creation.

I tried to absorb it, to keep this magic inside me.

Then, at noon, the voice of Monserrat Caballé singing *Ave Maria* poured into the vastness and filled it completely. Every note resonated in my gut and my throat. This was the first moment of joy I had experienced in the five months since the cancer diagnosis. I had not forgotten the cancer – the thought of it was lurking, even here – but for a few moments it was pushed aside by a soaring elation. Tears welled up and blurred the jewel-bright sunlight.

I was surrounded by genius and I was overawed.

We went to a section reserved for prayer and contemplation where no photographs were allowed. I knew this could not last – the sun could not stay at that angle for long, the music must finish, time was moving on, but as we sat in silence I thought how lucky I was to have had this hour, in this place, today.

We were staying in Barcelona's Gothic Quarter and between visits to the Joan Miró Foundation and the Picasso Museum I stumbled to the hotel and collapsed on the bed, my limbs so heavy I wondered if they would ever move again.

We booked evening meals in restaurants only four or five steps from the hotel, and even then, I wondered if I would make it.

We spent New Year's Eve in a Lebanese restaurant eating humus, olives and flatbread. To our right was a group of beautiful young women wearing high heels, applying lipstick, taking selfies. To our left was a bunch of handsome young men who drank tea from silver teapots and smoked shisha pipes that clouded the air. A singer in a white jacket set up a keyboard and sang passionately in Arabic as the beautiful women flirted with the handsome men; there was much smiling and calling and one of the women dashed to the men's table for a selfie. Midnight came and went, and it was not acknowledged by the crowd; no one seemed to know or care that 2018 had gone and 2019 arrived.

For me, too, the change in year was oddly insignificant because although the year of diagnosis had passed, the cancer experience continued.

Two weeks after returning from Spain I went for a check-up with the breast oncology consultant. It was a young woman doctor I had never seen before. I was disappointed. It seemed that whenever I saw a doctor I either misunderstood who they were (thinking I was seeing an oncologist when I was seeing a breast surgeon, or thinking I was seeing a breast surgeon when I was seeing a houseman, or thinking I was seeing a radiotherapist when I was seeing an oncologist) or I was expecting someone familiar, but, like now, it turned out to be someone I had never met before.

I think this must be the definition of 'multidisciplinary'.

I told this new doctor about the hot flushes, confusion, nausea, fatigue. She told me it was early days and as far as the radiotherapy was concerned, side effects were to be expected for up to a year. As for the tamoxifen, she tapped away on her screen and gave me the figures: *if* I continued to take the tamoxifen there was a 96 per cent chance that in five years I would not have died of breast cancer, there was a 90 per cent chance that in ten years I would not have died of breast cancer and there was an 83 per cent chance that in fifteen years I would not have died of breast cancer. The tamoxifen reduced the chance of recurrence by 30–50 per cent.

I was not sure I understood the statistics, but Cello was nodding. How I wished I had listened forty years ago to my A-Level Statistics teacher, Miss Levers, instead of chatting to the lad in the desk behind about Freddie Mercury. Now a bit of her knowledge would have been useful.

The doctor reiterated what the breast care nurse had said on the phone – if the side effects were unbearable, stop taking the tablets. But I told her I was too frightened to do that. I asked if she could give me something to counter the worst of the side effects – but she shrugged, 'That would be another tablet and another set of side effects.'

I felt abandoned.

For the sake of something constructive to say, I suggested I keep a diary of the symptoms and track if they improved. She agreed and gave me an appointment in four months.

I asked her, 'Why was I put on the type of HRT particularly associated with breast cancer?'

She replied, 'We don't put anyone on HRT here. You need to ask the people who did.'

Later, I phoned the NHS clinic that initially put me on HRT – the clinic with the reassuring grey-haired doctor – only to get a recorded voice telling me the number was no longer in use.

When I was nineteen I joined a big organisation and was taken aside by Ernie, another member of staff who was near retirement. 'You are very lucky to have this job,' he said, bending down, peering intently at me over his glasses, 'you have a gold-plated, non-contributory pension. Do you realise how lucky you are?'

I didn't. I found talk of my pension depressing and ridiculous and I wished Ernie would go away. I lasted five years in the job before escaping back to full-time education.

Thirty years later, the day before I discovered I had breast cancer, I received an annual statement from this pension scheme that was payable when I was sixty. I phoned them to ask about early withdrawal, imagining using it for a fantastic holiday, and was told the only way I could apply for early release and not lose out would be on health grounds, and I laughed, *I actually laughed*, because I felt so healthy. I look back and cringe. How privileged I was, and foolhardy and naïve, to believe that with diet and exercise I could control my health and my life. I jotted the words 'early release only on health grounds' on the pension statement and filed it away.

Several weeks and a cancer diagnosis later I dug out the statement and wrote to them. It seemed like a win/win situation – either I would be too healthy to get my pension early, or I would get my pension early. I suspected it would be the former – but it would be nice to be declared 'too healthy' in writing.

I was called for an assessment by an 'Occupational Physician' at a premises on George Street, the fancy shopping street in Edinburgh.

As I walked past the January sales in White Stuff, Jo Malone and Whistles on a cold morning I realised I was looking forward to it. I would be able to talk to a doctor for more than a few minutes about the experience of cancer. They may not be able to do anything about it, but they would have time to listen to me – the meeting was scheduled for an hour. I had a great urge to talk to someone who understood.

I was asked to wait in the foyer. The office was done up like a cheap spa with geometric wallpaper and what looked like TK Maxx mirrors and lamps. There were enormous chairs that infantilised, making me feel as small as Alice in Wonderland after the 'Drink Me' potion. Another middle-aged woman sat in the next chair and we found ourselves laughing and swinging round like a pair of kids at the office open day.

I heard a voice behind me: 'Catherine Simpson?' and I spun round. I steadied the chair and nodded. He was stern-faced and bald with something of the headmaster's office about him. I half expected him to say, 'Answer properly. Only donkeys nod.'

He introduced himself.

'I thought it would be a woman,' I said.

'Well there was a 50/50 chance,' he replied.

This was a man who dealt in probabilities.

I followed him through the disorientating building, along corridors, up and down stairs.

His office was vast with the atmosphere of a chiller cabinet. He sat behind his desk wearing several buttoned-up layers: shirt, waistcoat, jacket, body warmer. He apologised for the cold as I stripped off my coat and cardigan, down to a T-shirt, because my skin was burning.

I clutched my notebook, which contained a list of the symptoms I was living with. I outlined the dizzy headaches, the insomnia, the dragging fatigue, intense anxiety, depression and hot flushes, but when I got to the brain fog – the feeling that I was losing my memory and my mind – I burst into tears. I explained that sometimes I could actually feel a thought leaving my head – but I could not prevent it. Grim-faced, he leaned behind him and took a box of tissues off a shelf and put it in front of me.

He continued to tick boxes on the form with his silver ink pen. He asked if I had tried counselling and I said I had not been offered counselling. I felt I was having a conversation with some-one who was pretending to be a human.

After he had finished ticking his forms, he fitted the lid on his pen and placed it in its holder. He told me he would be in touch with my medical team for confirmation of what I had said.

As I left the building, I pictured him being switched off and put back in his box.

I wandered home, lost and empty.

A month later, I was copied in on a letter the doctor had sent to the pension company. In it he stated that 'Once the side effects have settled ... there is a hope that, within twelve months, Catherine will return to reasonable levels of fitness...'.

I was asked if I wanted to make any comments and I replied, 'Who is to say the side effects will settle? What if I don't return to reasonable levels of fitness. What then?'

To be told I was not eligible for my pension did not feel as satisfying as I had hoped.

I did not receive a reply to my questions, but only a printed form with the 'No' box ticked in black ink pen.

I lived on high alert. My eyes skimmed newspapers and online articles for the word 'cancer' in the way they used to do for the word 'autism' after my daughter was diagnosed fourteen years ago.

I was both drawn to and repulsed by the word 'cancer'.

When high-profile people died 'after a short illness' or 'after a lengthy illness' I searched the story for clues. Was it cancer? If the article didn't specify, I checked; were they treated at a cancer centre? Were there thanks to oncologists? Cancer charities? If so, my heart gripped and clenched; I felt a lurch, a tremor, a shift. That could have been me and I was embarrassed my first thought was for myself.

Twenty-Eight

It was three weeks until my book launch and it felt unreal and intimidating. How could our old family photo be the cover of a book? How could my life be a published story?

Wandering round the Scottish National Portrait Gallery, I noticed the people portrayed wore uniforms, insignia, medals, suits, robes, ruffs, ruffles, sashes, jewels, corsages, headdresses and capes. They were protected as surely as if their clothes and accessories were an exoskeleton. By contrast, a naked self-portrait showed the artist's red-raw knees, scrawny thighs, sagging breast tissue. How vulnerable he looked.

I needed my own exoskeleton.

The right clothes have always been a protection; the right shoes stopped me getting bullied at high school. My mother took us to be measured up for Clarks Startrites while we were at primary school but after that it was up to us – we chose what we liked, and we lived with the consequences. I arrived on the first day of high school in enormous platform shoes and never looked back. Through crippling 'granny shoes' to bouncy crepe wedges, I was happy to suffer to be fashionable. As a friend's Scottish mother said, 'You may as well be deid as oot' the fashion.'

'Sensible' shoes were anathema to me. For weekend wear I bought red and yellow shiny platforms in a cheap shop above Keenway supermarket. One day we went to a shop called Tommy Ball's in Blackburn with racks of shoes stretching across acres of carpet with the word 'Ball's' woven into it in red and blue. '*Ball's*' as far as the eye could see. It was a wonderland. The shoes had ankle straps and platforms and high heels. 'Patent leather,' I gasped; 'plastic,' said my mother. Anything was possible at Tommy Ball's.

High-heeled shoes were transformative, they were Cinderella's glass slipper and Dorothy's ruby slippers, they were glamour and elegance. There was nothing like the click of high heels as you walked to show you were grown up. 'You'll ruin your feet,' said my mother, but even a visit to hospital to see my aunt after she'd had her bunion shaved off didn't stop me.

I dreaded getting big feet, which seemed manly, ungainly and ugly, so I squeezed into shoes a size too small to try to contain them. Agonising ingrowing toenails, sore joints, blisters and painful mobility were worth it in this, my DIY modern-day version of Chinese foot binding.

Clothes were a disguise, a façade, a display, a demonstration of allegiance, a comfort, a confidence boost – so to prepare for my book launch I booked an appointment with a personal shopper at a department store on Princes Street, Edinburgh.

On the day, I was directed through the womenswear to a door hidden at the back, like *Mr Benn*, a cartoon character from the 1970s, who was transformed into a pirate, a spaceman or a cowboy simply by changing his outfit in a shop cubicle. Maybe this personal shopper could transform me into a confident writer ready to launch a book.

'You look like a woman who dresses for comfort,' the personal shopper said, and I looked down at my black jeans and T-shirt, mute.

I perched on a sofa beside a glass-topped table covered in copies of *Vogue* and admired some glittery dresses on mannequins stacked in the corner.

'Those are Christmas clothes, ready to be sent back,' she said, waving her hand dismissively, 'last season' – and she disappeared onto the shop floor.

She came back peering around a mound of garments.

'Oh, yes,' I said, spotting one or two black dresses. 'They look like the sort of thing I would usually wear.'

'Well, I'll get rid of them then,' she replied, 'you're here to find something different.'

She weeded out the black dresses.

'I want to see you in a jumpsuit,' she declared. I laughed nervously. Maybe I would emerge more *Josie and the Pussycats* than *Mr Benn*.

She encouraged me into red lace and green satin, pleats, wraparounds and zebra print until eventually we got to the black jumpsuit; it covered enough (the radiotherapy burns under my arm) and yet revealed enough (my undamaged cleavage).

I sashayed in front of the mirror.

It was the perfect exoskeleton.

I joined a creative writing course at Maggie's Centre. In the absence of counselling, writing with a group of people who shared my experience might help me put cancer into perspective.

But in the first class the course leader said the course was not to write about cancer and explained that participants may want to 'look outward and forward and beyond cancer'. Even as she said this, and I nodded along cooperatively, I knew I needed to look inward, to examine the experience of cancer. I had a lot of mental sorting and filing still to do. I may have been moving through it, but I was far from moving beyond it.

To show willing, though, I joined them in the garden with my notebook to study the first stirrings of spring. I noted the snowdrops and the cyclamen, the Lenten rose – as brazen as a child's plastic windmill – the blossom bursting on bare branches and the desiccated beech hedge ready to re-explode in green.

But it was impossible not to see it as a garden of cancer metaphors: the coiled ferns, small, apparently harmless, but invasive, hard to kill and capable of taking over the entire garden if left unchecked. And the newly planted trees, fragile and secured to canes to give them the support to thrive, which made me think of Cello bringing me here every day.

I peered to the right at the houses backing onto the hospital. Did living alongside a cancer unit make you feel safe, as though you'd taken out some sort of insurance? Or did you avert your gaze? Or grow accustomed?

But what really drew my eye was the view to the left, beyond the soothing plants and the outdoor ornaments, past the refuse containers and air-conditioning units and through the windows to the patients in the chemo ward lying on beds separated by magazine racks and bins of surgical waste. I studied their faces in profile, as they lay being poisoned to stay alive, as still and as silent as photographs.

The best thing about Maggie's Centre was that I was not the ill one, the medicated one, the flawed one, the pitiable one, the one who had got it wrong – because everyone here had cancer.

Elsewhere, cancer felt like an open sore that needed protecting, but at Maggie's that wound was accommodated. No one said, 'Are you over it now?' No one asked the wrong question.

Sitting at the central table you could chat with a stranger about scones one minute and mortality the next; from the weather or your holidays in one breath to night terrors or how easy it is to feel abandoned in the next.

But when I saw other people with their vulnerable, bald heads and their faces bloated with steroids, I knew their journey had been more brutal than mine. One lady told me I was lucky not to have had chemo, and seeing her yellowing, dried fingernails lifting from her nail beds, I hid my bitten nails under the table. I have picked the skin around my finger-ends and bitten my nails on and off all my life, and made them sore day after day, week after week. The sight of her painful-looking, gnarled fingers sent my overthinking into overdrive and I got stabs of both imposter syndrome (was my cancer bad enough?) and survivor guilt (why was I lucky enough to escape chemo?).

The weekend before publication, my publisher said there may be a review in *The Sunday Times*; the paper had asked for photos, but there was no guarantee, so not to get excited.

I was not excited, I was terrified.

I fell asleep on the Saturday night only to wake in the small hours with the familiar burning skin and feelings of terror, wondering how I could sleep again, even fleetingly, waiting for this possible review. What had possessed me to write the book? Panic flapped around the bedroom like a trapped crow. If only I could press Rewind. Abort. Delete.

I blinked into the blackness, eyes adjusting, and I picked up my phone. It was 3am. This was the witching hour for Google; the hour when I Googled everything I could think of about cancer; the loneliest, most remote hour when I had no defences.

Then I realised the review might already be online.

I lay in the darkness not Googling cancer for once but Googling myself – another indication if any were needed that life had spiralled into strange places. A link to the review popped up and I nearly dropped my phone on my face. I struggled to a seated position then froze, filled with dread, excitement, horror; the terror of finding out, fighting with the need to know.

Cello stirred: 'What are you doing?'

'There's a review,' I whispered, even though he was awake.

But the review was behind a paywall, so my eyes fastened onto the only visible words: 'In this superb memoir...'

The jangling cacophony in my head mixed with the heartbeats

echoing around my body, and from the chaos a thought emerged: *maybe* I will survive this.

Two days before the launch, I went to London to do some publicity organised by my publisher.

I was staying at the Bloomsbury, a hotel steeped in literariness in an area steeped in literariness. There were portraits of writers along the corridors: Wendy Cope, Jo Shapcott and Seamus Heaney, while Andrew Motion stood vigil outside my bedroom door.

I half-expected to see Mrs Dalloway heading out to buy the flowers herself.

I ate dinner on the Dalloway Terrace, which was festooned in wisteria and fairy lights and where the bill arrived, of course, inside a copy of *Mrs Dalloway*.

Being in this fancy hotel, a far cry from my usual Travelodge, had an unreal quality – like being in the Cancer Centre did. That feeling of *How did this happen to me?*

The bar was lush-red art deco, which I viewed over the rim of a G&T, savouring everything about it before signalling to the barman to bring another.

It was as though a cackling witch in a fairy tale was twisting together the good and the bad in my story, the dream and the nightmare, the blessing and the curse, and spinning them together until they were fused into one surreal life.

The next morning, I went to the BBC Radio 4 studios to be interviewed on *Woman's Hour*. The interviewer, Jane Garvey, bobbed around the Green Room beforehand, shaking hands. I asked her what the first question would be, and she said, 'I don't know.'

Later I waited beside her in the studio, breathing deeply, terrified I would get tamoxifen brain freeze live on air.

After the show, I told her about my fear of on-air freezing and blurted out, 'I've had breast cancer. I've been struggling.'

I don't know why I was compelled to tell her – maybe it was her kind and confiding manner or maybe it was because every time I told someone it diluted the news a little more. Whatever the reason, I was glad I had.

From being raised in a family that did not speak about difficult subjects, cancer appeared to have turned me into someone who could not stop.

My book launch was at Waterstones in a bright, airy space with a spectacular view of Edinburgh Castle. One of the usual questions asked of an author at a launch is, 'What are you working on now?'. We decided that my friend Sam, who was chairing the event, would not ask me that so I did not have to mention cancer.

But the final question from the audience was: Would I write more non-fiction?

The hours spent writing about life before and life after cancer over the preceding months flashed through my mind, my mouth opened and closed silently, and then I replied, 'Well, I've been dealing with a cancer diagnosis and I've been writing about that.'

Again, I was glad I had spoken the words out loud.

As I signed books at the end, a friend dashed over indicating my new outfit and squealed, 'Ooh, chemo diet!' I smiled and replied, 'No, Slimming World.' I was not giving cancer the credit for anything, let alone weight loss.

Nina was to marry her American boyfriend, Shane, in Las Vegas in June so we went to buy her wedding dress. She knew what she wanted, having seen it in a kilt-maker's window on the Royal Mile. I dragged myself out of bed, exhausted, headachy and dizzy.

Then I Googled myself (it had become a bad habit since the launch the week before) and I discovered a new review of my book in *Vogue*.

Thanks to my flattered writer's ego, I walked to the dress shop with a spring in my step. How powerful is good news and what a strong antidote it is to physical misery.

When I bought my own wedding dress twenty-five years ago it was only me and Mum in the tiny boutique and Mum was tired and ill with what would eventually be diagnosed as non-Hodgkins lymphoma. She slumped on a small gold chair gazing into the middle distance and said, 'I'm afraid you are on your own today' as I bought a dress that didn't fit.

I wanted to be more present for Nina.

Nina's choice was a full-length purple and blue tartan dress with a ruched skirt and laced-up bodice. It was a perfect frame for her tattoos, including the small red heart in her elbow ditch that said 'Mum'.

Twenty-Nine

Six weeks after the radiotherapy, I received an invitation to Breast Cancer Care's 'Moving Forward' course. If the robotic pensions doctor would not lend me a sympathetic ear, maybe this course would.

It was held in a 1970s hotel on the edge of town. I was early and joined the silent circle of other early birds still wearing their coats, hanging about outside the meeting room. We helped ourselves to coffee from a giant urn – the sort that never works until someone with the right touch manages to splutter coffee into the too-small cups – as we watched two ladies in bright orange logo T-shirts set up the room with an overhead projector and the inevitable forest of leaflets.

'It doesn't matter how early I am,' said one as she rushed past, 'there are always people here!'

Nobody talked. The corridor was ill-lit and oppressive. Had I made a mistake in coming? In the distance, Jackie Wilson sang 'I Get the Sweetest Feeling', but here in the corridor you could hear a pin drop. As a rule, I would have broken the ice and started a conversation but today I did not have the energy. There was a chair a little further along the corridor and I went and sat on it, apart.

I felt tearful, alienated and hugely self-conscious. Accepting that I had had cancer treatment, and that I belonged here at all, was an ongoing battle.

As we went into the meeting room, we were given sticky name badges. There were Susans, Karens and Julies – the names of women born in the sixties, names from my high school register.

A speaker gave us a talk about bra fitting. She passed around 'breast forms' – artificial breasts to fit into bras for women who had had mastectomies. They were heavy and dense and as we weighed and prodded them the dam broke and everyone started talking, asking about lopsidedness, underwires, swimming, beachwear. My alienation evaporated, and I was glad to be here with this group of women.

A nurse arrived from the Western General to talk about the after effects of radiotherapy. She was a young woman bursting with energy who looked no-nonsense, efficient, effective and not cancerous. Definitely not cancerous.

I assumed I was not the only person in the room who, post-cancer, was jealous of those who radiated energy and good health and the confidence it brought. I assumed I was not the only one who admired this woman's professional presence and remembered longingly to when I had had that too.

'Who has pain?' she asked. Almost everyone's hand shot up. 'Who has fatigue?' Everyone's hand went up.

She said the pain would probably be lifelong, but rather than this being depressing, it was empowering to be told the truth like a grown-up. She acknowledged many of the problems I had – tiredness, skin discoloration, itching, shooting breast pain and nagging shoulder pain – and this was validating.

The group let out a collective breath. Our experiences were real. It was rare to encounter such honesty, and both devastating and strangely comforting when we did because at least she was giving it to us straight. There was no flannel here.

We each received a tote bag of free gifts. Even in these circumstances, a tote bag of free gifts is a cheering thing. It contained a pink notebook, a pink pen, a pink water cup for the gym and a pink fan. There was also something called a 'Chillow Pillow' to help you keep cool at night.

I went home and watched a YouTube video about how to activate my Chillow Pillow. The video had been made by a woman at once mumsy and little girl. She bustled about a kitchen somewhere in the United States, filling the pillow, perversely but correctly, with hot water, wearing a red T-shirt with *HAPPY* written on it. She was earnest, keen to help us fill our Chillow Pillows, as her white cat surveyed us from his scratching post.

She mesmerised me. Below the video was the comment: 'Jesus, this video was mind-numbing.' But I watched her several times.

What was the fascination?

I think it was the comfort of shared experience, and the feeling that this unknown woman understood and *cared*. The video had thousands of views, so it wasn't just me. She may have been a continent away, but when she lay her pony-tailed head on the pillow and her round, plain face gazed beseechingly into the camera and she said, 'So, yeah, I'm going to try to get a good night's sleep on my Chillow', I wanted to cheer and cry at the same time.

It was late March and Cello was keen to go away for a few days. Again, I was daunted by the energy it would take and a knot of anxiety formed in my stomach at the prospect of airports, transfers, queues, long walks, getting lost, being a hostage to life at someone else's pace.

We flew to Krakow. My holiday reading included two library books: the first a memoir by a woman in her forties with breast cancer. She was rich and wrote of going to America to get brand-new treatments – cutting edge, 'right at the limits of knowledge' – and of her experiences in London private hospitals. She had a sense of humour, a light touch. During the flight I became fond of her. The book ended on an optimistic note as she laughed with her children.

On arrival in Poland I Googled her to discover she died shortly after writing the book.

That was a kick in the teeth.

My other library book was about someone declining traditional cancer medicine for a range of alternative treatments: detoxing, coffee enemas, vitamin injections, cutting out dairy, cutting out sugar. I went timidly to Google to do a search, and yes, she was dead too.

I was sick of this.

I threw the books back into the suitcase. The only other book I had with me was *The Cancer Journals* by Audre Lord.

Instead, I watched reruns of *Frasier* on Netflix.

The following day I woke with red welts across my chest from trying to scratch a deep unscratchable itch in my radiated right breast as I slept.

We wandered around this city of spires and towers, turrets and finials, vast squares, endless archways and soaring stained glass and I realised in the evening, when I returned to the hotel, that despite the pain, itching and tiredness, for a few hours that afternoon, for the first time since the diagnosis almost eight months before, I had completely forgotten cancer.

The creative writing course at Maggie's Centre finished so I signed up for a journalling course. I have written diaries intermittently for years and have a compulsion to buy notebooks, so I was keen to attend, but the real reason was that I was not ready to let go of Maggie's.

I did not have to let go, of course; there was no time limit on how long I could use the facilities, but I didn't want to 'drop in'. I wanted the full-blown commitment of being on a course. I wanted the comfort of the big table, the welcoming faces, the feeling of camaraderie with the other participants, the sense of belonging and purpose.

Our tutor, Val, suggested a list of journalling tools: notebooks, pens, glue – and I felt joy at the prospect of virgin stationery, like

I had when my mother handed me a new pack of felt pens and a drawing book at the beginning of the school summer holidays forty-five years ago.

Val described various types of journals – travel, birdwatching, gardening through the seasons, food, cooking. She suggested doodling, drawing maps and collaging and a frisson of excitement at this freedom to create rushed through me. She got out bright green paint and dolloped it in our journals, handed us wooden sticks, and told us to play with the colour and within minutes the group had created images of trees, fairies, ships, planets and exotic birds.

We decided to write gratitude journals. Val said studies showed the practice of gratitude could lead to a healthier, happier life. I didn't care *which* studies showed this; I was happy to take this information at face value because it felt right to decide to be grateful. The thought of creating a gratitude journal was already making me sit up straighter, concentrate harder and begin to hum with life.

We were asked to write: 'What I am grateful for here and now...' and our pencils flew across the pages. *I am grateful for Maggie's, for this journalling course. I am grateful I have a fan bought in Spain. I am grateful I went to Spain. I am grateful for my warm coat and my bus fare. I am grateful for our flat, the fridge of food, the burning candle on the table, the news channel, the coffee machine. I am grateful for cheese scones, Jaffa Cakes, chicken curry and slow cookers. I am grateful for the creativity of others, all the art galleries within walking distance and the inspiration they hold, I am grateful for Netflix and books; all the books I own, which I will not have time to read even if I live to be a hundred...*

Searching for bright spots was compulsive and heading home on the bus I scoured the free newspaper for things to be grateful for: a man rescuing an eight-stone sheep from a cliff face; a tortoise called Mikey being fitted with a GPS after more than one hundred escape bids...

As I went through the day I searched for the good, the beautiful, the unexpectedly pleasurable, often things so small they would previously have gone unremarked, and I wrote them down. *Spring bulbs in a roofless chapel, pineapple upside-down cake, the cat asleep in a perfect circle, librarians, podcasts, Lara's texts as she travelled around the US, sunshine on Calton Hill, Nina's home-made cherry pie, my dad's new hearing aid, impromptu prosecco with the neighbours...*

When friends visited, I asked them to fill in the journal, too, which they did with greater or lesser enthusiasm: *A pint with Kev ... a new bed ... strawberries and cream ... Chihuahuas ... sunshine ... Sugababes on Spotify ... aquaerobics...*

Sometimes I found myself gripping the edges of the journal like one of those polystyrene floats from childhood swimming lessons, as if it was the only thing stopping me from sinking.

I was silenced by the number of middle-aged women who said what they were most grateful for was HRT.

Many days I struggled to be grateful; when my head was fuzzy from lack of sleep, when life was one overwhelming flush after another – several each hour lasting minutes at a time, merging into each other – when they possessed me and trapped me in a body I still didn't recognise as my own.

One day I lay on the bed, every muscle aching. I knew I must stop worrying about the effects of treatment. I decided to take a few minutes out, shut my eyes. I flicked on the radio. A medic was being interviewed. A 'vagina doctor' apparently. She was batting away myths about the female sex organs, dealing with the worries of the listeners: no, you shouldn't have to endure very heavy painful periods; no, you don't need over-the-counter vaginal preparations; no, there is no limit to the number of times you can take the morning-after pill. Then the presenter read out: 'Why has my clitoris disappeared? I have had breast cancer and been on tamoxifen for several years and I think my clitoris has disappeared.' The presenter remarked, 'Can your clitoris really disappear?' And the vagina doctor hesitated, not batting this one away, 'Er, well, long-term use of certain drugs can affect the architecture of the body and how it reacts...'

There was no escape from this subject. I turned the radio off and curled into the foetal position.

Six months after having surgery in the Breast Unit I visited my friend, Eileen, on a medical ward in a different part of the hospital. I was struck by the contrast with the Breast Unit – the lack of cushions and comforts here, the absence of what used to be called 'a woman's touch' that had been evident in the Breast Unit.

My friend was wrapped in a fleecy dressing gown, sitting in an armchair, alone in the visitors' room. Beside her was a table with a sign: *Table Broken. Condemned.* The television was switched off and had its own sign: *In Loving Memory of Isa.* There was a trolley of worn-out books: *Healing with Angels*, *Hymns Old and New*, alongside paperbacks with peeling stickers: *3 for 1 Great Value Summer Sizzlers*, and jigsaws of vintage cars and thatched cottages.

My friend, looking pale and drawn, ate a white meal from a tray. Her sandwich was pure white: white bread, white butter, white filling. She ate it deliberately, delicately, and when she had finished, she lifted the lid from a polystyrene pot and peered in at some pure white rice. She shuddered and put the lid back on.

I leafed through *Hymns Old and New* and found a yellow Post-it note stuck inside with a list of what appeared to be selected funeral music, written in a quavering hand: RAF March; Hymn

49, 'Be Still'; Hymn 311, 'How Great Thou Art'; Hymn 405, 'The Lord Is My Shepherd'; and, at the end, written in shaky capital letters; Hymn 109, 'DO NOT BE AFRAID'.

Thirty

Despite loving playing outside as a child, I knew nothing of organised 'leisure'; Dad did hard physical work for thirteen hours a day then fell asleep in his armchair. Adults having the time or the desire to walk for fun was incomprehensible. As kids, we viewed ramblers using the public footpath through our farmyard as intruding weirdos in kagouls. My sisters and I used to gather to point at them and stare them away.

I also knew nothing of organised sport – my village primary school was too small to create a team of any kind – but me and my best friend Alex spent every playtime leapfrogging, skipping or walking in never-ending circles with our arms around each other's waists (although we were warned never to do this once we got to high school in case they thought we were both 'one of them').

The primary school headmistress, Miss Proctor, was an elderly lady with more interest in embroidery than PE, so the only physical education we got was 'Music and Movement' – a BBC radio broadcast in which a posh woman instructed you to 'find your own space' and then 'grow like a tree' or 'flutter like a leaf'. This was a little dull; the only excitement was when Cousin John crashed over like a great oak in a high wind, which was impressive.

However, my relationship with exercise did not deteriorate until high school games lessons and the sheer uncomfortable, self-conscious awfulness of it all; the hockey on icy playing fields with bare legs and arms, the Aertex tops, the hypothermia, the hockey being called off only 'when it was too cold for the sticks', the 'bullying off' (in which my little sister lost a front tooth), the compulsory netball, the macho jostling and shouting: *Pass! PASS!* The 'tennis' with saggy-strung racquets, the fruitless search for lost tennis balls, the threats that if you 'forgot' your kit you'd do it in your knickers.

Things changed after leaving school with the advent of the cult of aerobics. Cult leader, Jane Fonda, dressed head to toe in Lycra and accessorised with sweatbands and legwarmers, demanded we 'Go for the burn', telling us 'No pain, no gain!' and assuring us that 'Discipline is liberation'. From 1982, *Jane Fonda's Workout Book* was on the *New York Times* Best Seller list for two years.

Hyper-energetic aerobics was something I could get on board with because it promised to 'reshape', 'sculpt' and 'shrink' my body, which fitted in perfectly with my obsessive calorie counting. It was another way of taking control. When I felt guilty about that second packet of Batchelor's Savoury Rice, I would go to Slim Jim's Health Club and do not one, but two aerobics classes back to back, not taking a break even when I felt the semi-digested rice trying to crawl back up my throat.

In 1993 I joined yet another gym, this one located in an Edinburgh city centre hotel. Using the equipment was not exercise for the joy of it, nor even for the health of it – as evidenced by the fact I caught the bus the 500 yards there – it was exercise to look good on my wedding day. Nevertheless, it was boring. One day I spread the *Daily Mirror* on the handlebars of the exercise bike to read the celebrity gossip while I pedalled, but after twenty minutes I'd still only used up half a Twix.

The boredom was spectacularly broken only once, during the New Zealand rugby union tour of Britain, when I went for my after-workout jacuzzi to discover it full of All Blacks. (It takes just three All Blacks to fill a hotel jacuzzi.) I sat beside the pool pretending to read my newspaper, watching them watching me.

I exercised out of guilt – feeling lazy if I didn't – I exercised out of a never-ending desire to improve my body, to achieve something, although I'm not sure exactly what would have satisfied me. Even when I took up tap dancing and enjoyed the spangle and the make-up and the step-ball-changes, I still managed to turn the class into a surrogate slimming club by taking my scales along every week and getting everyone to weigh in.

Pre-smartphone, I wore a pedometer and walking without a tracker counting my steps became a 'waste'. I resented any step taken and not tracked. *I could never get those steps back.*

There was an unbreakable link between movement and weight. Fitness equalled slimness.

The only exception ever had been yoga. Following my failure at school sports, this was something I could do, and enjoy doing. My hypermobile joints made me good at it. Yoga was quiet, calming, non-competitive and, most importantly, my teacher, Martina, did not shout.

Three months after my hospital-based treatment ended, Macmillan Cancer Care offered me exercise classes for people who have had cancer. I went along and was asked about my goals. I told them my goal was to be strong again. And for the first time, I realised I wanted to do aerobic exercise to be strong not slim.

They asked how I was coping emotionally: 'How confident are you that you can cope with whatever happens to you?' And I realised that was what cancer had taken away from me and what I was trying to recover – the belief that I could cope with whatever happened to me.

There were people in the class ranging from their thirties to their eighties. Some of them had been fit before cancer, while others looked like exercising was new to them. Some were wearing yoga pants or gym shorts, others looked like they'd nipped out to do a spot of shopping.

There was a line of blocks down the middle of the room, for balance practice. We warmed up standing in a circle around them; *Heel toe! heel toe!* shouted the instructor and we obeyed as the Bee Gees sang 'Stayin' Alive' and we looked for all the world like the

1970s teenagers a lot of us once were, at the disco, dancing round our handbags.

There was a circle of chairs, each with an activity assigned. We moved from chair to chair – a minute and a half each at 'wood chops', 'bicep curls', 'hamstring curls', 'side-steps', 'squats', 'hand to knees'.

Hayley, the young woman who ran the class with style (wearing full make-up and a small blonde beehive), selected the music and we lifted and bent and stretched to T Rex's 'Telegram Sam' and Neil Young's 'Heart of Gold'.

'I wanna live…'

The only one in the room not singing was Hayley.

'I don't know it,' she shrugged, 'but when I put this stuff on it goes down well.'

I smiled and kept singing and side-stepping.

'…and I'm getting old.'

'Layla' by Derek and the Dominos came on and the opening riff whipped me back forty years. For a few seconds I was not fifty-five in an exercise class for people recovering from cancer, I was back in the farmhouse kitchen aged fifteen with a drunken boyfriend arriving on his moped after closing time at the pub. 'I've brought your record back, Café' (he could never say 'Cathy') and the seven-inch single of 'Layla' crashed from the bottom of his leather jacket onto the lino. I was remembering the drama of being fifteen and mad about a boy my mother couldn't stand, when 'Layla' was unceremoniously cut off. 'No!' a grey-haired lady and myself shouted – both of us obviously ripped back from the past to the here and now.

'Well, it goes on a bit, doesn't it?' said Hayley.

The room had glass walls on two sides. The view was of trees, vivid green with new leaves, and as I sang and moved to the music, I felt a soaring optimism.

Macmillan also offered three sessions of complementary therapy for cancer patients. Complementary therapy (treatment used alongside traditional medicine, not instead of it) is believed, among other things, to help patients relax and gain a sense of control. The Macmillan centre was in the Western General, next to the Breast Unit – not a place I really wanted to revisit – but as I turned off the heavy-duty industrial corridors of the hospital into the Macmillan unit, I realised this was a place apart and the atmosphere lightened.

There was a view of their small garden in which everything was decorated – metal butterflies were affixed to the wall, a grinning clay tortoise climbed up a planter, a bird house swung in the buddleia, glass globes and wind chimes dangled from every branch, a wooden robin had its feet nailed to the decking.

If there was a bright side to be found, these people would find it and attach a novelty to it.

The tiny garden was surrounded by high walls that shut out the rest of the hospital. I complimented them on their pots of lavender and marigolds. 'Some of 'em are plastic!' a man replied cheerfully. There was a strong sense of a deliberate attempt to cheer, to put on a brave face.

A circle of volunteers drank tea round a table laden with chocolate biscuits and a box of fruit, with a sign stuck to it: *Guess my Weight*.

I had entered a cocoon.

I was offered three sessions of the Bowen technique – something I had never heard of – but the atmosphere of the place gave me faith. Helen, the therapist, had a kind face and a gentle voice. I lay on her massage table fully clothed, which was a relief after all that stripping off for radiotherapy, as she made gentle rolling motions with her hands on my back and legs. She gave me a tissue soaked in 'Unwind', a blend of lavender, sandalwood and frankincense essential oils, and put on a tape of birdsong, waves, pan pipes and piano.

It was hard to believe these gentle-as-air touches were doing me much good, but I left each session smiling and emotionally lighter.

Another therapist, Moira, gave me breathing and visualisation techniques to help me cope with the hot flushes. She said to move slowly when the burning began, to help quell the sense of panic. We talked about accepting that it was happening; breathing deeply, reacting slowly, waiting for it to pass, to experience the entire sensation as a moment-by-moment mindfulness exercise. What a relief to be told to stop fighting myself, to stop railing against my own body, to accept reality and let it be.

Was I finding my sea legs with this new life? I tried to convince myself I was.

In May I was back at the out-of-town 1970s hotel for another 'Moving Forward from Breast Cancer' course, during which one nurse had the unenviable task of telling this roomful of terrified, jittery women what to be on the lookout for in case there was a recurrence of the cancer.

She checked more than once: did we really want to know? Yes, we said, we really did. She clearly didn't want us searching for symptoms where there were none, but eventually advised us to be aware of bone pain, weight loss, a persistent cough, headaches and increased tiredness.

I wrote it down and underlined it.

The course leaders explained that in effect this course constituted the other half of our treatment, so that once the medical treatment (surgery, chemo, radiotherapy, hormone therapy) had been organised, and the 'safety net' of the hospital had gone, we did not feel abandoned and alone.

They said patients were often left confused, wondering why they weren't celebrating – and I remembered the emptiness when I saw the *After Radiotherapy: What Now?* leaflet balanced on my clothes in the empty treatment room.

A visiting psychologist explained that time often froze at the point of diagnosis, that the world carried on, but the person with cancer was stuck, unable to move forward.

We collectively nodded.

We shared so many experiences, these women and I: the tiredness, the shock and disbelief, the sense that we should not talk about it any more in case people were bored of cancer or considered it 'all in the past', and the consequent loneliness and resentment this caused. Every time these subjects came up, the room burst into animated chatter, everyone swapping stories with a sea of understanding faces and nodding heads.

Cancer generated a comradeship, an understanding, a shared, unforgettable experience that bonded this group of disparate women.

I received an email from a local hotel offering *Spa Treatments for Those Living with or Recovering from Cancer.* The email was illustrated with a dimly lit picture of an orchid beside a religious-looking statue. The treatments on offer had names like 'Soothe and Nurture' and 'Catch the Breath'.

I was offended.

Was it coincidental or did they know about my cancer? If they knew, how did they get my email? Was it a scam? Why did I need 'special treatments'? Why couldn't I get normal treatments?

In a fit of pique, I phoned to demand an explanation. I could not get through: *I am sorry. All our operators are busy.* I listened to ever-lasting 'Zorba the Greek'. I was cut off, twice, and became overwhelmed by hot flushes and frustration. More 'Zorba'.

Eventually I got hold of someone who explained their therapists had been trained on 'where and how to massage' after cancer treatment. She explained that if you have had lymph nodes removed (which I had), incorrect massage could lead to lymphoedema – a lifelong problem that caused swollen limbs.

Was this true? If so, why was I discovering it from a receptionist at a spa that I had phoned out of anger? I thanked her and backed out of the conversation with as much grace as possible.

Shortly afterwards, a cancer charity asked me if I would volunteer to be massaged by therapists training to treat cancer patients. So, the spa was right.

I agreed to be a guinea pig.

The training was on a Sunday afternoon in yet another out-of-town 1970s hotel. The lady arriving ahead of me – another guinea pig – announced she had had a tumour on her leg – 'Very rare!' – so I was compelled to say, 'Breast Cancer, nothing special'.

There were eighteen therapists working on nine cancer patients all in one big conference room separated by makeshift screens. One of the two therapists assigned to me saw me glancing around. 'It's all women,' she reassured me, as we both caught sight of a man in the corner. 'Well, except him, and he's…' she waved her hand, '…over there.'

I got undressed under a towel, in the style of a 1950s sunbather, with two therapists forming a towel-tent around me.

I stuck my face through the hole in the massage table and gazed at the brown and maroon geometric carpet and I heard the room falling silent around me. As the massages began, I reflected that this, a communal massage with complete strangers, was yet another cancer experience, something else unexpected that had been brought my way by cancer.

I read about 'forest-bathing' – the idea that spending time around trees was good for mental health – so I jumped on the bus and headed down to the Royal Botanic Gardens in Edinburgh, which has 70 acres of landscaped gardens, ten glass houses, a rock garden, a Chinese Hillside, an arboretum, a pond and apparently 70,000 plants. I wandered the gardens, which were bursting with blossom and rhododendron buds, making sure I touched the trees, resting my palms against their trunks.

It was a peaceful place, but I was not at peace as I became increasingly obsessed with the memorial benches that lined the paths. I read each plaque on each bench with a lump in my throat. *W GORDON SMITH 1928–1996, FOR MY DASHING HUSBAND WHO SWEPT ME OFF MY FEET TO A ROLLERCOASTER LIFE OF HAPPINESS. TOGETHER ALWAYS. JAY.* (Written all in caps like someone unfamiliar with the internet.) And others ... *Emma Louise, A beautiful and beloved friend, daughter and wife... Margaret & James, Together again...*

But worse, I focused on the dates, doing lightning calculations of how long these lives were – as though that would indicate my own life expectancy, some kind of minimum lifetime guarantee.

I needed to stop and left the gardens in a hurry.

Shortly after my trip to the Botanics, I saw photographs of a friend 'forest bathing' in Finland in which she, her husband and son were lying face down on the forest floor with their noses in the moss.

Clearly, I had been doing it wrong.

I carried a fan in my handbag. As soon as I started on tamoxifen, I knew I needed a fan to help with the overpowering heat surges. I bought several fans in Spanish souvenir shops – lace fans, sequined fans, fans painted like an English canal boat. I had them all over the house, on every table, in every bag but I still felt self-conscious using one in public. No one else in Scotland appeared to need a fan.

I am sure Glenn Close in *Dangerous Liaisons* gave all sorts of messages with her fan: *Meet me in the boudoir, I need you, I want you, I love you.* The only message I gave with mine was: *Please do not stare, I am burning alive and trying not to panic.*

Lara gave me a large white electric fan to put beside my bed. It stood there like an angel with three wings. I couldn't work out why it made me uneasy, until I remembered an identical one standing vigil beside my mother's deathbed in the melting summer of 2006.

Thirty-One

In the months following the diagnosis everything was about cancer.

The constant narrator in my head repeatedly reminded me I was a woman who had had breast cancer, and wove everything – television programmes, newspapers, books – into my cancer narrative.

I even saw cancer when it was not there, clicking on an article 'The four stages of cancer' only to start reading about 'The four stages of a career'.

I was role playing in a live action game.

I scanned the people around me to work out how they fitted into my cancer story. What had these strangers to add?

At a charity ball in a hotel under a motorway bridge in Glasgow it took me a few minutes to realise Cello and I had been seated with the entertainment and the politicians. Across the table was a middle-aged man called Raymond who was bald and bespectacled and said he was booked to sing covers of Adele, Avicii and Coldplay.

I was not sure how Raymond fitted into my cancer story, but to my right was an accountant turned hypnotherapist, and he was a possibility. I told him about my cancer – I was unable to stop myself – and asked if he treated people for anxiety. He told me about Thought Field Therapy and gave me a quick lesson in tapping the forehead, temples, under the eyes, chin, chest, underarm, between the ring and little finger. He swore by it. Said it helped alter negative moods.

A troupe of young girls in Lycra started dancing, flinging themselves about the stage, doing handstands, cartwheels, star jumps while we tapped away: forehead, temples, under the eyes, chin, chest, underarm, between the ring and little finger. 'Keep tapping,' he said, 'keep tapping.'

After we finished tapping, he introduced me to Ricky, one seat along. Ricky was wearing a kilt – in fact, full Highland dress – and he passed along his business card: *Spiritualist Medium and Psychic*, which showed a blue eyeball close up, not unlike an ad for cataract removal.

I told him I had seen his booth in the hotel foyer, next to the bottle tombola, festooned in velvet with a hand-drawn sign in pink glitter: *Fortune Telling, Ten Pounds*.

Perhaps Ricky could look into my future and tell me I would live to be old? That would be worth ten pounds.

He sighed. 'Am no' a fortune teller,' he shook his head. 'I dinnae look into the future. I pass on messages from the other side.'

He was agitated about the velvet booth and the glittery sign. 'I cannae work in these conditions,' he said, 'I need quiet.' He left the dining table to go and sort out his ambience. I shouted after him to put me on his waiting list – never mind that he did not tell fortunes – maybe he would be able to tell me *something*.

A couple of hours later, after we had finished the honey-roast ham and raspberry cheesecake, I was escorted upstairs in the lift for a consultation with Ricky. He was working from the entertainers' dressing room and had placed a gold dining chair amid piles of tulle and neon nylon. Around the room was the detritus of a hundred dancers: discarded tights, scattered make-up bags, tins of hairspray.

I perched on the gold chair and Ricky stood in front of me, one hand on the brass buttons of his waistcoat, the other hand aloft, finger pointing skywards like an aerial. He closed his eyes to tune in to 'the other side'.

Ninety per cent of me was treating the experience like theatrical entertainment, but the other 10 per cent wanted so hard to believe. He took deep breaths; his head dropped onto his chest then lifted again like a dog catching a scent.

'I've got a Margaret and another lady, younger ... your generation. Are they somebody?'

'Yes,' I replied, 'it could be...' I was about to explain they sounded like my late mother and late sister.

'No! Don't tell me. Just a yes or a no. A yes or a no.'

'Yes.'

His nose was in the air again as he listened intently.

'The younger woman is very animated. She's doing all the talking. She says you've recently done something you've wanted to do for a long time and never thought you would.'

I took a deep breath to tell him about my memoir.

'Just a yes or a no,' he said.

'Yes.'

'You should be very proud, the younger woman says, very proud indeed.'

I was again conscious of wearing the right mask and I smiled as though messages from my dead family were commonplace – but my scalp fizzed.

He frowned, 'I've got a Bert ... is that somebody?'

'No,' I said apologetically.

'Herbert? Robert? Hubert? Just a yes or a no.'

'No.'

Ricky continued to tune in, finger aloft, eyes shut.

'I'm getting the Beatson ... the Beatson...'

I hesitated. I knew the Beatson was the Glasgow Cancer Centre, but it was not the one I had been going to.

'...someone's been going to hospital?' Ricky said.

'Yes'

'I'm saying "the Beatson" but by that I mean any cancer hospital. Somebody's been going back and forth to the cancer hospital?'

'Yes.'

'Well, these ladies – Margaret and the younger one – they say it's all over now.'

I gulped. 'Yes. Right. Thank you.'

'I'm getting a Maureen ... a Maureen...'

I racked my brains, desperate to find a Maureen. I didn't want to let Ricky down now; my Grandma was a Marjorie, did that count? Then reluctantly, 'No.'

There was a lot more, but it was hard to remember the details afterwards because 'Margaret and the younger one' reassuring me the hospital visits were over had drowned out everything else.

Walking back into the ballroom, I felt I hadn't so much been in the dancers' dressing room as on another planet, somewhere not quite real, like much of my life over the previous year.

A friend told me, 'You have been heroic throughout!'

According to my *Oxford Paperback Dictionary*, 'heroic' is showing the attributes of a hero, and a 'hero' is a *man* admired for his brave or noble deeds.

I did not feel heroic and considered this as I wandered around the Scottish National Portrait Gallery, a place like the Vue Cinema where I could escape my life and peer into other people's.

I wondered what being 'heroic' meant. Did it mean not making a fuss? Keeping calm and carrying on? Keeping trauma hidden – behind closed doors, in your head?

The 'Heroes and Heroines' exhibition in the gallery informed me that Thomas Carlyle proposed the creation of this portrait gallery 'for the celebration of heroes', which he saw as 'those who represent their age in an exemplary way and would serve as models for future generations'. He apparently believed that 'personal integrity was the basis of heroic action', which would manifest itself through 'seriousness, courage and hard work'.

I drifted from portrait to portrait. There were, it seemed, many ways to be heroic: you could build a lighthouse. Be 'zealous in your Scotch Evangelical faith'. Speak at anti-war demonstrations. Use your oratory to win a war. Be a member of the Bloomsbury Group. Build schools for 'the ragged'. Be the butcher of the Somme. Be the Tsar of all the Russians. Be at the Queen's left hand. Or according to the poem 'Invictus' by William Ernest Henley, paraphrased on the gallery wall, 'Be master of your fate and captain of your soul'.

There were women here, too. Queen Victoria, of course – three depictions, in watercolour, oils and marble; literally stony-faced. Also Flora Clift Stevenson, an educationalist and philanthropist; Caroline Norton, a social reformer; Fanny Stevenson, a writer and wife of Robert Louis; and Mary Somerville, a scientist and mathematician. Although when Carlyle originally suggested this gathering of heroes it did not include women – their sphere was domestic, where polite society expected them to be the 'angel in the home': dutiful, submissive and self-sacrificing.

I studied a portrait of writer John Wilson, who was described as: 'A larger than life character ... upright, knocking down, poetical, prosaic ... hard drinking, fierce eating, good-looking, honourable and straightforward.' And I wondered: who would be a heroine when you could be a hero?

The final face in this pantheon of heroes was a fresh-faced young man who, in 'just under 13 days' in 1881, was the first to cycle from Land's End to John o'Groats on a penny farthing.

Heroism seemed to include an element of choice – choosing to do something difficult, often to benefit someone else, whereas I had had no choice to make and had been flung into a situation in which I had at times been terrified, resentful, self-pitying, angry and needy, and the only person who benefited from all of the medical care and attention was me.

There were many ways to be heroic, and I doubted that as a cancer patient I had been any of them.

Having cancer had made me sensitive to the remarks of others, but how could I expect people to know what cancer was like if they had not lived it?

I considered myself empathetic, believing I would not say the wrong thing to someone in a crisis – but one day, while running a writing workshop for young people, I realised I too could be staggeringly dense.

I had set a writing exercise inspired by the phrase 'I dream of…' and I read out my own scribbled example:

I dream of packing a bag, buying a ticket, and never coming back. I dream of never-ending journeys on boats, buses and trains. I dream of being able to fit everything I own into one bag and carrying my world with me.

These 'dreams' were presumably inspired by my desire to leave cancer behind and start again, but as I read them out, I remembered that, unexpectedly, we had been joined in the class by a young Syrian refugee. What must she be making of my 'dreams'?

I was mortified and decided that, in turn, I must be more understanding of people who, without malice or cruel intent, blundered into saying the wrong thing about cancer.

I returned to the Cancer Centre for a review of the tamoxifen, having been on the drug for seven months. I took along my diary of symptoms – a long list of sleepless nights with constant hot flushes, insomnia and getting up as tired as when I went to bed, followed by depressed, anxious days.

I told the oncologist I might be coping a bit better, and she asked whether this was because I felt physically better or whether I had adapted and learned to live with the symptoms, and I nodded, yes, mainly the latter. I was acclimatising to a reduced quality of life.

I glanced at my notebook of questions (a more businesslike one this time, not the silver cracker notebook) and I asked, 'Does "positive thinking" make a difference as to whether the cancer comes back?' I glanced up and we looked at each other and then both of us burst out laughing. When we stopped, I said, 'So, not at all then?' And she shook her head. 'No, not at all.'

People asked me, 'Are you in remission?', 'Are you cured?', 'Have you got the "all-clear"?' And yet no doctor had ever used any of those terms.

I asked her, 'Do I have cancer or am I cured?'

She explained that some cancers do come back and that she could not guarantee mine would not be one of them. The surgery had removed the tumour and the radiotherapy was designed to kill any remaining cancer cells, then the ongoing tamoxifen was there to stop any random cancer cells from thriving; nevertheless, they could not be sure that the cancer would not return, because some traces of cancer could have remained that were too small for current tests to reveal.

This was not the black and white reassurance I craved.

She said, 'You had cancer in your body; now – as far as we know – it has gone.' She looked at me. 'That's all we can say. The cancer has gone, as far as we know.'

Summer was coming and my skin looked milky pale, but I could not risk getting a suntan because of the sensitive skin caused by the radiotherapy.

'Get a spray tan,' someone suggested.

This was another first, another 'cancer experience', I reflected, as I stood naked, bar tiny pants, in a makeshift tent in the back room of a beauty parlour, as a therapist, gowned, masked and gloved, sprayed dye at me as though she was painting the back bedroom.

Up and down. 'Turn! Keep still!' Up and down.

When she finished, she left the room, giving me instructions to stay still. She set an alarm clock. It was cold. I was naked, and as I stood there, barely breathing, watching the clock ticking down the ten minutes, I had a horrible flashback to the freezing, naked, stillness of radiotherapy and I vowed I would never do this again.

Thirty-Two

On a warm summer night, I went to see Kylie playing against the backdrop of Edinburgh Castle with its ring of flaming torches. I had bought the tickets at my lowest ebb seven months before because fourteen years ago, Kylie had had to cancel Glastonbury due to her breast cancer diagnosis and yet this year she was back there in the 'Legend' slot.

She stepped from a mirrored box onto the stage, a fizzing bundle of energy and charisma in a white spangled jumpsuit. She sang and danced for an hour and a half: all of the old hits, some new ones, five costume changes and no let-up in pace. She did not appear to be a woman whose life had been made small by breast cancer – on the contrary, she glowed, she laughed, she joked, and she did the whole thing in five-inch gold stilettos.

I wondered how many other women in the sell-out crowd had experienced breast cancer and were here to watch Kylie like a talisman, like a singing, dancing charm bringing us all good luck.

A lot, I suspect.

I watched her performing, looking gorgeous, and I remembered my fears of the anti-oestrogen drug 'turning me into a man' when what I had meant was it would make me less feminine, somehow neutralised. Watching Kylie, who has herself taken tamoxifen, I realised that for me femininity is a performance, aided by props. It is a state of mind, an illusion, a choice. Femininity is more than oestrogen.

It was not up to tamoxifen how feminine I chose to be – it was up to me.

I wanted the Kylie concert to be a happy ending – a line drawn a year post-diagnosis, a see-how-far-I've-come moment, but I was thwarted.

We were helping my daughter's American husband apply for a British visa and were faced with the horror of dealing with the Home Office: contracted-out services, impenetrable websites sending us in blind circles, £5.42 to send an email, contradictory information, overnight rule changes, the impossibility of speaking to a human being, spending fifty-odd pounds to courier documents only to have them returned within days with a note saying, in effect, *Nope, not here*, haemorrhaging money as the time ran out to submit supporting documents.

I watched my daughter's mental health wobble and I cried down the phone to our MP and our immigration lawyer – a man who was already drowning in other people's despair: 'I've got a Pakistani woman here who needs two thousand pounds by tomorrow or she gets deported...'

Tension was painfully high; there was so much at stake, and every day the faceless, intransigent bureaucracy got worse.

The Edinburgh International Book Festival was in full swing and most days I spent time in the authors' yurt in Charlotte Square, just because I could. I had an author's pass and was making the most of it, spotting celebrity authors, chatting to writer friends, being where it was all happening in August for book lovers. There were contacts to be made, acquaintances to meet, friendships to develop – a chance to feel like I was part of it all.

The trouble was, I felt on the edge of losing myself. I felt disconnected from everything around me; I could feel my mind unravelling; my speech had speeded up – or at least I think it had – my thoughts crashed and collided; I overshared my worries about the Home Office visa with people I hardly knew, I couldn't stop. They were kind. They sympathised, but inside my head there was a tiny voice – the voice of the pre-cancer 'me', the old me, who was still hiding behind the dustbin in the garden of my mind, watching the chaos being wrought by cancer and its treatment – whispering, 'Stop it. Go home. You shouldn't be here.'

Then, one day, after another Home Office dead end, I found myself bent double in my office chair at home, head in hands clutching my hair. I had the urge to drop to the floor and curl into a ball. A postcard by my desk read: *Let each moment happen*, an exhortation that made sense once, but not now – not when every moment was agony.

There was a skewering from my throat down to my stomach and my breathing was shallow. With each Home Office knockback, my stress levels had risen and now I was back in an out-of-control world where I was helpless and powerless. It was as though I had rewound a year to the dizzying, terrifying time of cancer diagnosis – the time when I may-or-may-not have had cancer, which may-or-may-not have spread.

I thought I had been dealing with this cancer thing, but it seemed I had not.

Despite all of the complementary therapies, the support groups, the gratitude journalling, the exercise classes, the healthy eating, the yoga and the determination, I felt the accumulation of a year of fear and the lack of agency it had created.

I felt the weight of the final straw.

That night, lying in bed awake in the blackness, I thought, 'I can't cope. I hope the cancer comes back.'

I have had bouts of depression since before I had a word for it. As a young teen, there were times when a heavy bleakness smothered me, making the world a stagnant and dead place, blacking out all hope or point. I told no one. It never occurred to me to, and I wouldn't have known how to express what was happening to me if it had. I spent a long time sitting on my bed staring at nothing.

I eventually consulted a doctor about my mental health for the first time in my mid-twenties after I had walked around a supermarket feeling that the supermarket was unreal and I was unreal, convinced I could see myself doing the shopping. An out-of-body experience near the kitchen roll.

In those pre-Prozac days, I was prescribed my first antidepressants, big purple pills, whose name I probably never took in. These were pre-internet, pre-easy-access-to-information days and I had no idea what they were or how they worked, but the very act of having them in my hand helped. I stayed on them for six months, and the depression lifted, but I still told no one.

The second and third times I took antidepressants were for postnatal depression after each child.

Again, there was that feeling of unreality, of hearing a baby crying and not knowing if it was happening. Day by day I acted the part of the new mother, wore the coping mask, smiled, told no one except Cello, aware that I would be judged.

Then ten years later, another depression that would not lift. 'You'd better get to the doctor!' said Cello, finding me sitting at the kitchen table staring blankly into space. More antidepressants.

Many people are suspicious of antidepressants. Fear and shame swirl around them: the fear of being left in a dulled state, the baseless fear of becoming addicted, the shame of having 'failed' in needing them at all and of not having tried hard enough to 'pull yourself together', the shame when people accuse you of thinking a tablet can solve everything, of not dealing with the root cause of the problem.

Antidepressants have been good to me. I am not anti-medication – despite HRT being the probable cause of my cancer – but it still took the wish for the cancer to come back to make me realise I had to go to the GP for help, that I was all out of other options.

He was a GP new to the practice, with a passing resemblance to the angel Gabriel, or maybe that was just me. The relief at being heard was immense. He was the kind of doctor whose presence was curative; like the complementary therapists, he reassured merely by being.

He did not dismiss me with the assertion that 'another tablet, another set of side effects' like the oncologist had, but said 'the kind thing to do' was to put me on a low dose of antidepressants.

I was so overwhelmed by his understanding that I started crying in his consulting room and as he lunged for his box of tissues, I remembered the long line of other medics and therapists over the past year who had lunged for their tissues in their consulting rooms.

I knew the medication *would* come with its own side effects, but I was willing to try anything to stop feeling like a stranger to myself.

The side effects kicked in immediately – a distancing, a fuzziness, a dry mouth. Three days later I had my own event scheduled at the Edinburgh International Book Festival, which had been a dream for years, and I knew I had to do the best acting of my life.

But a miracle also happened: straightaway the antidepressants stopped the worst side effects of the tamoxifen – the vicious burning flushes and deathly chills that I had endured day and night for almost a year stopped. I dreaded it being a mistake, a temporary anomaly, but it didn't seem to be. They had gone.

On the day of the book festival event there were 200 people in the tent. The antidepressants made them feel at a great distance, as though I was looking through the wrong end of a telescope. White noise and echoes filled my head. I was dizzy with occasional waves of nausea – yet I had to read and talk and answer questions on stage as though my mind was sharp and alert. I constantly sipped a glass of water so I could talk despite my dry mouth.

The audience was warm and receptive as I balanced along this wobbly mental tightrope.

I wanted to confide in them about my antidepressants making this a surreal experience, but even though I was there to talk about, among other things, breaking the stigma around mental illness, I did not mention it. Would I embarrass them? Would it be unprofessional?

I wish I had had the courage to be more honest.

Within a fortnight of starting the antidepressants, many of the remaining tamoxifen side effects had gone, as well as the violent temperature changes, the depression, the endless circling anxiety, the hopelessness and the sleeplessness.

I had been released from the tamoxifen prison.

In addition, the antidepressant side effects had faded. Nothing in the outside world had changed: the Home Office was still intransigent, I was still one-year post-cancer diagnosis, but because of the antidepressants, everything in my head had changed.

It was like meeting myself last year.

Cello and I were walking near the travel agents and went in to look again at Faisal's map. The two feet of blue ocean that separated us from Buenos Aires now seemed traversable in a way it had not a year ago.

'Let's book it,' I said.

The boundaries of my world were re-expanding.

Thirty-Three

Scrolling through the photos on my iPhone, gazing at images from before and after 1 August 2018, the day everything changed, I look the same, but I am a different person.

Before cancer I lived like I had a guarantee of *something*.

Now I know we have a guarantee of nothing.

Cancer has been a process of unlearning.

Cancer made me vulnerable, as though my mind and body had been peeled and left raw, open to the elements, unprotected. It made me reflect on how I had treated my body over the years and how newly grateful I am for it. Of how I have worried about being too tall, too small, too fat, too buxom, too hairy, too pale, too flabby. I had ignored, abused and taken my health for granted and fallen into traps about what a woman should look like, act like, think like – what a woman should *be*. Cancer made me reassess everything and be grateful for this one body I have to live in.

Cancer forced me to face my own mortality. Death stopped being something that happened to other people – or to me at some far-off time or place. For a while it became a force beside me, edging into the next seat, its thigh rubbing mine, its arm brushing mine, its breath on my face.

When I next hear death stir and clear its throat – whether that is sooner or later – will I be calmer? I suspect not. Like Old Mary, I will probably always want a little bit more.

Fear of cancer lurks below the surface. When I read of author Elizabeth Wurtzel's death from breast cancer, on the anniversary of the completion of my hospital treatment, I recalled the oncologist saying, 'The cancer has gone, as far as we know. That's all we can say', and I felt a numbness creep down my arms and my heart begin to race. I was slipping into panic mode so easily – until I took some deep breaths and it faded.

That was life now.

A year ago, cancer taught me I was not who I thought I was.

I was someone who got cancer at fifty-four.

I was not 'cool' with the idea of death.

I was not always the strong one, the brave one, whose job it was to help other people. I was sometimes the one who needed help.

The voice in my head, narrating my story, went haywire. It became hysterical. *I am not me! Am I anyone?* Thoughts swirled round like scummy water going down a plughole.

I had to reset my identity and in doing so I discovered I could accept help.

I discovered I had lived with a false sense of security – the belief that I could control my health and my fate – when real life is more random, less predictable, than that.

I discovered that life does not end with a cancer diagnosis, but life-as-you-know-it might, at least for a while.

I discovered that underwired bras are little better than whale-bone corsets and life is too short to be trussed up.

I saw for the first time that the obsessive worry, guilt and shame around food that had wasted so much time and energy over the years was disordered thinking; that food is a friend not an enemy, a source of pleasure and nourishment, not of stress and panic. That the aim in life cannot be to die thin and hungry. That the craving for the smallness and tautness of prepubescence, when life was less complicated and I felt that I could fly, was a lost battle to say the least.

For the first time, I took aerobic exercise to grow stronger, not to get thinner; to be healthy, not to look good. I was interested in what my body could do, not only what it looked like.

For the first time, I wanted the privilege of ageing healthily, not ageing 'youthfully' by trying to deny the ageing process. I realised 'body confidence' does not mean 'feeling thin and attractive' but means being able to think about something else entirely. I didn't want to hear any more about fifty being the new forty or sixty being the new fifty. Every year, I was a year older and that was a gift.

Cancer made me slow down and be grateful.

Cancer made me speed up and get things done.

Cancer made me live intensely in this one body of mine.

At first, cancer made me feel diminished, but I am not less; I am everything I was before, plus all this.

I am remade; grateful for the opportunity to rethink my body and my life, to keep living, to keep learning.

Afterword

In Summer 2019 I attended a meeting of 'cancer survivors', where a nurse said, 'You probably want your old life back, your old selves', and I whipped out my notebook to write down her secrets because, yes, indeed, I did want my old life back.

'You probably want your "old normal" back,' she went on, then shook her head, 'but you can't have it because it's gone. Your life has changed for good. The old normal will not come back and you need to work on creating a "new normal".'

I tried to absorb her message. It was the first time I had heard the phrase 'new normal', but nearly two years and a pandemic later, it is commonplace.

In early Spring 2020, when we were put into lockdown to control the spread of coronavirus, I watched as the entire country appeared to experience its own cancer diagnosis.

There was the shock and disbelief that we were facing a pandemic at all, but especially that it could *happen to us*. This kind of catastrophe happened to other people.

As with my cancer diagnosis, normal life vanished overnight. Simple pleasures were out of reach. Straightforward tasks became difficult. Buying basic groceries, getting fresh air and exercise took forever. A fear of the unknown and the future hovered. The unfortunate became ill, some chronically so. The most unfortunate died or were bereaved.

Life pre-coronavirus seemed long ago. Vanished.

As with the cancer (at least for those of us in lockdown as opposed to key workers facing the dangers of the virus every day), there was a sense of unreality, an other-worldliness. The outside world became distant, and close family all important. We were trapped in our own bubbles, gazing out, listening to the birds. Even in the city centre you could hear the birds, as weeds sprouted between cars parked in front of shuttered shops.

As with the cancer, hair became an issue – but this time not whether I would lose it, but whether I could face going grey, and I discovered that yes, I could; it wasn't grey but silver and I liked it.

As with the cancer, there was a surreal sense of time standing still, of fearful waiting. And a fury that it had happened at all. 'I'm sick of it! I wish it would all just go away!' I heard someone say. Well, yes. Fury is a part of grief and grief does not manifest only after a death.

As with the cancer, the fear of the virus's return was real, a lurking worry. Would COVID-19 always hover in the back of our minds? Would we ever regain that carefree ability to jump on a plane, or would we adapt and learn to live with its presence among us?

As with the cancer, there was a deep unease that life had changed forever. We had to acknowledge that a world we had once taken for granted could disappear overnight and become unknown, and if it had done it once, it could do it again.

As with the cancer, there was a dawning realisation for many that although the pandemic hadn't killed them, it had left them weakened through lingering after effects.

But as with the cancer, there was also a sense that perhaps some changes were for the better. The break with reality created by COVID also created freedom from the tyranny of the 'shoulds' and 'musts' and 'oughts'. *I must go to … I should visit … I really ought to…*

We who are reading this are all pandemic survivors of one kind or another, not something we ever thought we would be, but a title we have attained nevertheless. Few have been left unscathed by illness, loss, fear or trauma, but we are the ones who got through. Millions have died of COVID-19 worldwide since 2020, and many millions more have been lost to cancer, as they are every year. We are the ones fortunate enough to have another go at life, putting into practice the lessons a pandemic taught us. We are the ones with the opportunity to be flexible, adaptable, to wear the world differently, and to not only survive but thrive. We have the time to work out what we want and need, not what we should ... must ... ought to want and need. Although we are also the ones who know we can guarantee nothing but this moment right here, right now. We are the ones who can still listen to the birds.

The trip to Buenos Aires was cancelled, of course, but I am still one of the very lucky ones.

'And now we welcome the new year. Full of things that have never been.'
Rainer Maria Rilke

Acknowledgments

Thank you to everyone who has lived parts of this story with me: family, friends, acquaintances, thank you all.

Special thanks to:

Staff at the Scottish Breast Screening Programme and the
    Western General Hospital Breast Unit & Cancer Centre.
Macmillan Cancer Support
Breast Cancer Care and Breast Cancer Now
Maggie's Edinburgh
Dr Christopher Stewart, GP extraordinaire.
My lovely agent, Joanna Swainson of Hardman & Swainson.
Sara Hunt and the team at Saraband – it's been a pleasure to
    work with you.

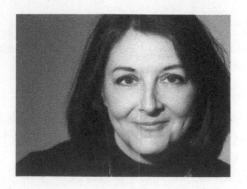

Catherine Simpson is a novelist, journalist, poet and short story writer based in Edinburgh. Her memoir *When I Had a Little Sister* was published by 4th Estate in February 2019, and her debut novel *Truestory* was published by Sandstone Press in 2015. In 2013 she received a Scottish Book Trust New Writers Award for the opening chapters of *Truestory*. Her work has been published in various anthologies and magazines, published online and broadcast on BBC Radio. Born on a Lancashire dairy farm, she is now based in Edinburgh.